MERIDIANS

of related interest

The Spark in the Machine
How the Science of Acupuncture Explains the Mysteries of Western Medicine
Dr. Daniel Keown M.B. Ch.B., Lic.Ac.
ISBN 978 1 84819 196 9
eISBN 978 0 85701 154 1

Sun's Dance of the Channels
Understanding Channel Interactions and Holography
Jonathan Shubs
Illustrated by Christina Malouf
ISBN 978 1 83997 223 2
eISBN 978 1 83997 224 9

Sun's Season of Channels
An Introduction to Chinese Philosophy, Chinese Medical Theory, and Channels
Jonathan Shubs
Illustrated by Fergus Byrne
Foreword by Simon Becker
ISBN 978 1 78775 902 2
eISBN 978 1 78775 903 9

The Acupuncture Points Functions Colouring Book
Rainy Hutchinson
Forewords by Richard Blackwell, Angela Hicks and John Hicks
ISBN 978 1 84819 266 9
eISBN 978 0 85701 214 2

The Acupuncture Point Functions Charts and Workbook
Erica Joy Siegel
ISBN 978 0 85701 390 3
eISBN 978 1 78775 009 8

MERIDIANS

Maps of the Soul

MIKE MANDL

TRANSLATED BY JOHANNA SCHUSTER

CONTRIBUTING EDITOR: HELMUTH SANTLER

FOREWORD BY DR FLORIAN PLOBERGER

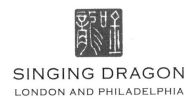

SINGING DRAGON
LONDON AND PHILADELPHIA

Originally published in Austria in 2020 by BACOPA
First published in Great Britain in 2023 by Singing Dragon,
an imprint of Jessica Kingsley Publishers
An imprint of Hodder & Stoughton Ltd
An Hachette UK Company

2

Foreword copyright © Florian Ploberger 2023
Front cover image source: Felicitas Grabner www.felicitasgrabner.com

A CIP catalogue record for this title is available from the
British Library and the Library of Congress

ISBN 978 1 83997 671 1
eISBN 978 1 83997 672 8

Printed and bound by CPI Group (UK) Ltd, Croydon, CR0 4YY

Jessica Kingsley Publishers' policy is to use papers that are natural, renewable
and recyclable products and made from wood grown in sustainable
forests. The logging and manufacturing processes are expected to conform
to the environmental regulations of the country of origin.

Jessica Kingsley Publishers
Carmelite House
50 Victoria Embankment
London EC4Y 0DZ

www.singingdragon.com

Contents

Foreword by
Dr Florian Ploberger

Dear reader,

'Our task in life is to become the person we are.' May this quote, attributed to the Indian lawyer and resistance fighter, revolutionary, publicist, ascetic and pacifist Mahatma Gandhi (2 October 1869–30 January 1948), make us aware that we are inherently healthy and complete. We have simply forgotten it. There are numerous paths to reclaim our true potential, to get healthy. Reading this book is one of them.

In recent decades, Traditional Chinese Medicine (TCM) has seen a tremendous boost, both in China and in Europe, Australia and the United States, where a host of practitioners now offer various methods of TCM. How did this come about?

It all started in 1972 when Richard Nixon was the first American president to visit the People's Republic of China. The media spread images of an acupuncture demonstration, especially organised for the president and his entourage, which roused the interest of the scientific community. The various methods of TCM were presented to the visitors from the US in several different hospital wards. The visitors were particularly fascinated by open-heart surgery performed with acupuncture anaesthesia.

The previous year, the journalist James Reston accompanied the American table tennis team to China in preparation for the presidential visit; while he was there, he suffered acute appendicitis. On the front page of the *New York Times* of 26 July 1971, he reported his experiences of the successful post-operative analgesic treatment with three acupuncture needles.

In 1997, during a study trip to Beijing, I was able to participate in a caesarean section at the same hospital visited 25 years previously by President Nixon and his team. The mother received acupuncture anaesthesia.

Since the 1970s, numerous excellent textbooks on the methods of TCM have been translated from Chinese and others written by Western authors. Many Chinese physicians have travelled outside China. In addition, many Western people have studied in China and deepened their knowledge of acupuncture.

Mike Mandl's book is concerned with the subject of the meridians as maps of the soul. After a fascinating introduction, the meridian systems and the most important acupuncture points are presented in great detail and in a completely novel way. The book offers a plethora of wise and insightful thoughts that inspire self-reflection in accordance with the words of St Thomas Aquinas (c.1224/25–7 March 1274), an Italian Dominican monk and one of the most influential philosophers and Catholic theologians in history: 'Health is not a condition, it is a mental state.'

I am delighted that Mike Mandl, someone I personally value greatly and whom I visit in his function as Shiatsu therapist time and again with much gratitude, has succeeded, on top of all his other activities, to publish this book with so much commitment, joy and passion for detail. Mike writes in an inspiring style, with many metaphors and much wisdom. His writing has depth yet is easy to read.

At this point, I would like to quote the author with an excerpt from the introduction:

> For those who haven't had much exposure to TCM and the meridians, this will be exciting new territory. It is my hope that therapists of a wide range of backgrounds will find this book helpful in adding to their knowledge and deepening their work.

I am convinced that you, dear reader, will thoroughly enjoy this book!

I'd like to conclude with a little story. The following ancient anecdote from the history of Tibetan medicine has been passed down over many generations.

One day, a teacher endowed with extensive knowledge – it was Jivaka, the Buddha's physician, whose Tibetan name was 'tsho byed gzhon nu – asked the students gathered around him to leave the classroom and search the vicinity for plants that had absolutely no healing properties. Furnished with this instruction, the students went forth.

One of them returned only a short time later. She carried in her hand a variety of roots, fruits from a tree, flowers and so on. Others took a bit longer. But one particularly gifted student couldn't find a single plant without healing properties, however much he tried. He returned empty-handed three days later. Of course, his teacher praised him, since, according to his teachings, nothing in nature is without healing properties. No matter whether it's a part of a plant, a Shiatsu treatment or a good book.

May reading this book bring you much pleasure and many insights!

With cordial wishes,
Dr Florian Ploberger

PART I

MERIDIANS: MAPS OF THE SOUL

Chapter 1

Meridians as Guides

The Search for All-Encompassing Wellbeing

We feel that even if all possible scientific questions be answered, the problems of life have still not been touched at all.

Ludwig Wittgenstein

'Health is a state of complete physical, mental and social wellbeing and not merely an absence of disease or infirmity.' With this definition from its Constitution, worded in 1948, the World Health Organization (WHO) followed the aim of detaching health from a purely biomedical view, considering health not as a given and fixed state but rather as a balance that is constantly renewed and actively created, which affects all areas of our lives. Decades later, we are further from this goal than ever before. Why? Have we not accomplished so much since then? We enjoy a standard of living unique in the history of humankind. We can draw on an excellent medical system and outstanding social achievements. We are looking at continuously rising life expectancy. We have freedom, leisure time and opportunities on a grand scale.

Yet, or precisely because of this, the all-encompassing health envisaged by the WHO seems to be present in only the rarest of cases. Rather, across the board, we are inundated with a plethora of new disorders and diseases. Many of these have their causes in the psycho-emotional realm or are related to lifestyle. Burnout, allergies and metabolic disorders are rising rapidly, even in the young and very young. The cost to the health sector amounts to billions. Is there an end in sight? Not in the foreseeable future. The fact that so many people suffer from a perceived lack of true wellbeing has resulted in a negative spiral, constantly exacerbating existing problems. We are hurtling with great speed towards a sick health system.

There are many reasons for this. Crucial aspects are certainly the increasing complexity and multi-layered challenges of Life 2.0. Added to these are affluence, weariness and exaggerated expectations: 'We want it all and we want it now!' Even worse: 'We can get pretty much everything – and now.' However, we're paying a high price for leading such a completely imbalanced life. Living a truly fulfilling and balanced life is a challenge that is difficult to master in this age of permanent availability, compulsory flexibility and gradually declining stability. Strictly speaking, we are continuously diverging from the emotional, physical and social wellbeing envisaged by the WHO, rather than getting closer to it. We are aware that something isn't right. We are aware that something is lacking – and we're searching for it.

But this search is not easy. The multitude of signposts for health and happiness are confusing rather than beneficial and supportive. What do we do when we feel a twinge in our bodies? What do we do when the soul hurts, when the mind is tired? There are specialists everywhere, accomplishing marvellous things. That's wonderful when there are specific problems requiring specific solutions. However, when it is about the bigger picture, about wellbeing embracing the entire person, then such a fragmented approach is not very effective. Whether of a physical or emotional nature, most problems are the result of an imbalance of body, mind and soul, of lifestyle and living conditions, as well as our desires and expectations of life.

A human being is a multidimensional being, a complex entity that is much more than the sum total of its functions. A human being is a dynamic system that is in a constant relationship and exchange with its environment. A lively balance, integrating all aspects of our life, is the best foundation for an all-encompassing feeling of health which includes personal growth and self-actualisation.

If we want to establish this kind of balance, we need an approach that will put the right tools into our hands. Among the various approaches for building bridges between body and mind, one truly stands out: Traditional Chinese Medicine, or TCM for short. Why?

Because TCM has defined health similarly to the World Health Organization – albeit 2000 years earlier.

In TCM, health means living in accordance with one's natural disposition and one's environment; an inner balance mirrored externally; an all-embracing sense of wellbeing and growth. In a nutshell: a fertile balance on all levels. Examining this topic over the millennia, TCM was able to develop and refine it further. This has led to the accumulation of unique knowledge, and its application in the world's most populous country has stood the test of time a zillion times over. Its success is, and will remain, valid proof of TCM's approach to health.

The system of TCM is strongly oriented towards immediate practical benefits. It can be instantly applied in everyday life. This is because the foundations of TCM – and in particular the theory of the meridians – are surprisingly easy to understand. Centuries of contemplation and practical application have led to the clarity of true understanding. By means of the meridian system, not only are we able to gain knowledge and insight concerning ourselves, our society and our wellbeing, but we can also take more responsibility for and proactively shape our lives according to our wishes. Constantly and actively creating and recreating this balance is not utopian. It is certainly achievable. This is also the wish and goal of this book.

The Meridian Principle: Making Life Run Smoothly

Imagine a wheel – a classic bicycle wheel with spokes. When all spokes are tightened evenly, the wheel runs smoothly. If, however, just a few spokes are too loose or too tight, the wheel wobbles. This has far-reaching consequences. The imbalanced spokes impair the smooth running, and over time various components will suffer one-sided wear and tear. In the long run, material fatigue may occur, and the affected spokes may even break. So it is better to be off to the workshop straight away to balance the wheel before it is too late.

In TCM, there are twelve main meridians. You could imagine the meridians as the spokes of a wheel and your life as its hub. When the meridians have a balanced relationship with each other, life will run smoothly and provide the foundation for health and wellbeing. But if there is an imbalance among the meridians, the same happens as with the wobbly wheel. Our life no longer runs smoothly, neither for us nor within us. Complaints of a physical or emotional nature may develop. They arise due to friction, fatigue or even the collapse of individual components. In this case, too, a quick trip to the workshop is recommended to get rebalanced. Even better, of course, would be regular maintenance to avoid problems occurring in the first place. It's much better to prevent illness than have to treat it. This is the approach of TCM: the common physician treats illness after it occurs, the superior physician before it manifests. A well-balanced wheel allows us to roll easily, swiftly and contentedly through life without having to put in unnecessary effort and without losing energy through unnecessary friction. That is one aspect of the meridian principle: maintaining and, if necessary, re-establishing health and vitality through continuous balancing.

Then there is the bicycle itself to be considered. A bicycle is there to be ridden. Life exists to be lived. With a well-functioning bicycle, we can gather speed; we can venture on ambitious trips and head for peak experiences. We can reach formidable goals. We can realise our dreams: health, vitality and a fulfilled existence – the goal of TCM. This is almost identical to the idea of health as all-encompassing wellbeing formulated by the World Health Organization 2000 years later. The meridian principle provides us with the key to reach this goal. But what actually are meridians? And how can they contribute to a smooth and even wheel of life?

Tracking the Meridians: How to Understand Them

Imagine the following situation. You're returning home from a journey late at night. You're tired and hungry, since what the airlines serve these days as a main course leaves as much to be desired as the leg room in economy class. You throw your bag in a corner, make a beeline for the fridge and take stock. Perhaps you're lucky and, despite your hasty departure, it harbours not only the foul smell of mould but also a couple of pleasant surprises. Okay, after a week's absence, the remains of the vegetables have seen better days, and a few other items seem to have developed a life of their own despite the overdose of preservatives contained in most foods these days. At least the smoked ham looks acceptable. But better be on the safe side and cautiously guide it to your nose. The odour test delivers what the eye had hoped for. The stomach approves the result with a demanding growl. Together with the emergency ration of crackers, you come up with a passable midnight snack. Done and dusted.

Eating: a completely normal everyday procedure with a logical order. Looking, smelling, chewing, swallowing, digesting. A completely normal process requiring many parts of the body to cooperate with each other and interact in a well-orchestrated manner: eyes, nose, teeth, tongue, chewing muscles, oesophagus, stomach – they all form a functional community for the purpose of food intake. But before we even get to the point when we target and devour the desired titbit, there has to be a stimulus, a need to be satisfied that initiates the entire process. It may be hunger, our mood for food or the desire to fill the terrible emptiness of a broken heart with calories. Whatever triggers the stimulus, it encourages us to carry out the relevant actions, one after the other.

To begin with, we check with our eyes to see whether the object of our desire lives up to our wishes or requirements. This could be while shopping in the supermarket, rummaging through the shelves in our pantry or harvesting in our garden. Then it's the turn of our nose, our olfactory sense, an instrument as archaic as it is powerful, with a subtle yet decisive influence. This influence is not quite as subtle if something is rotten – for example, bad eggs, or fish that is as far removed from being fresh as from its last encounter with the sea. A delicious aroma, on the other hand, will make our gastric juices flow, and we look forward to guiding the first bite to our mouth with relish. The nose determines whether what we have chosen visually will indeed land in our mouth.

Once the olfactory okay has been given, chewing can begin. Chewing not only adds to a more or less tongue-flattering experience of taste but is also the beginning of digestion. The bite is sufficiently crushed, ground and mixed with saliva – the more, the better. Only then will it be swallowed. The stomach further breaks down the food (bolus) received from the oesophagus in order to make it more accessible for the other digestive organs. If we were to mark and connect with a pen all the areas involved in this process, we would have sketched the first section of the stomach meridian.

Meridians Are Embodied Life Principles

For more than 2000 years, meridians have been the foundation for countless successful treatments with TCM – millions of them. Millions of times it has been empirically proven that the practice of TCM holds what its theory promises. Meridians are much more than dubious energy pathways. But nor are they precisely defined lines that cover the body and are studded with acupuncture points. This representation, while certainly being very descriptive, has little to do with the original idea of meridians. The mechanistic depiction of meridians is an artificial product of the Chinese cultural revolution, which reformed, standardised and structured the vibrant knowledge of TCM in order to convey the impression of a precision that corresponds to the ideals of science. On its journey West, a fair number of mistakes regarding translation and interpretation were added to the mix, and suddenly the image of the meridians was reminiscent of muscles and bones, along with clear tasks concerning the organs. However, it was never intended that way. Meridians are not abstract energy channels; nor are they precise supply pathways. Meridians are much more.

Take the stomach meridian, for example. Its pathway is no coincidence, and it's not abstract in any way. Its pathway comes about of its own accord and follows an inherent logic: it connects all muscles, structures and sensory organs related to a particular function. It is the blueprint of a goal-oriented entity. It stands for a principle expressed by the body: registering food, taking it in, processing it.

In TCM, however, food is seen as providing us not only with fuel on a biological level but also with everything else our body needs so that we don't feel that something is lacking. The principle of the stomach meridian is therefore not limited to purely physiological tasks. It also encompasses psychological and emotional aspects. Who hasn't experienced an unpleasant situation that upset their stomach and affected their appetite? Surely you can remember an event or a person that turned your stomach? Or have you ever had to chew a problem over? Has there ever been something that left a nasty taste in your mouth? Of course, these are just idioms, but they express the experiences and wisdom of many generations: that there is a close and direct connection between eating and our emotions, between our head and our gut. Or, put even more generally, that there is strong correlation between body and mind, between the physical and the emotional realm.

Isn't it the case that we somehow have to register, process and utilise everything we take in from our environment, be it information, sensory perceptions, feelings, thoughts or encounters? And doesn't this registering, processing and utilising represent the same process as the intake of food? And isn't the nutritional value of a steak the same as that of affection? So that inspiring people can satisfy us in the same way as a slice of cake?

Our heart, our mind and our soul depend on nutrition in the same way our body does. They rely on some means to keep them alive. Interestingly, the German word for 'foodstuff' is *Lebensmittel*, literally meaning 'a medium or stuff for living'. Without food, we will live in want; we will wither, emotionally and mentally. We need love, we need enthusiasm, we need a meaning in life. We hunger for it. We're looking for it. We're trying all kinds of different options until we find what fills us and makes us content. We need appropriate meals for all levels of our nature. Otherwise, and despite a full tummy, there will remain an inner emptiness.

Psyche (mind) and soma (body) are inseparable. They form an entity and are in a constant exchange. The meridians are the bridge clearly and explicitly expressing this connection. It's the stomach meridian's task to establish a balanced fullness in all areas of our life. The question is: What kind of nutrients do we have to ingest on the different levels of our existence in order to be really content? This is the stomach meridian's life principle.

Each of the twelve main meridians of TCM represents such a life principle. It is these principles that help us to act responsibly and proactively for the benefit of our health and personal growth. They can support us to reach our maximum possible potential according to our individual disposition. If we manage to establish a balanced relationship among the twelve meridians and their corresponding life principles, our wheel of life will run smoothly.

Energy: Effectiveness from Within

The foundation of TCM is the principle of yin and yang. Each pole has its counterpole. Yin and yang, day and night, summer and winter, heat and cold, south and north, birth and death, poverty and wealth, women and men. As far as our way of life is concerned, we should be aware that the external world of phenomena is complemented by the inner world of thoughts, convictions and emotions. In TCM, the outer world has a yin character. It is more stable, more constant and firmer. The inner world has a yang character. It is more fleeting, more variable, less tangible. The outer world is the realm of matter. The inner world is the realm of energy.

A major part of the problems in today's society can certainly be traced back to a strong focus on the outer world. We value material success more than inner success. We revere palpable status symbols more than a calm mind. Visible wealth is deemed more valuable than deep contentment. We willingly let ourselves be fooled by appearances and neglect simply being. We separate yin and yang. According to TCM, problems always arise when yin and yang are no longer in dynamic balance. Therefore, if we really want to get closer to genuine wellbeing, we should give our inner world of energy more space and more meaning.

The word 'energy' derives from the ancient Greek language and comprises the syllables *en* for 'inner' and *ergon* for 'to operate'. Energy thus refers to operating from within. We can easily observe this principle in our everyday life. When you are tired, you have no energy. But when you're well, you're bursting with energy. Some people tend to be energetic; they're real bundles of energy. Other people rob us of our energy. Some activities drain us of energy; others stimulate us. We can feel energy. We can experience energy in a very real and concrete way. Of course, this is also to do with our hormonal balance, our metabolism, our cardiovascular system and biochemistry. But that's only a part; it's certainly not the whole story.

Let's assume, after a day that was as long as it was strenuous, you are sitting completely exhausted in front of the television. You are incredibly tired; your eyes are heavy. You're dozing off again and again. Still, you don't want to miss the lottery results. A triple jackpot is on the horizon. You're holding the ticket in your hand, and it takes a great effort not to fall asleep as the numbers are announced. And then, with each figure appearing on the screen, you feel more awake. At the first one, you were just smiling a little, the same with the second. But at the third one, you were suddenly wide awake. From one moment to the next. At the fourth, your heart started beating faster. At the fifth, you broke into a serious sweat. And at the sixth, you collapsed. Because they were your figures. Jackpot.

You couldn't sleep the entire night. Your digestion was going crazy. Diarrhoea, accompanied by slight nausea, and your pulse never dropped below 100. Despite all this, the next morning you are full of energy and want to go to the newsagent as early as possible to make sure that your lottery ticket is indeed the ticket for a new life. But hang on: where is the ticket? Again your heart is racing, again you're breaking into a sweat, but this time it's about unadulterated panic. You're looking everywhere – once, twice, three times. And all over again. No ticket. You take your apartment apart. No ticket. You spend the entire day searching. No ticket. At some point, late at night, you break down with tiredness and cry about your cruel fate. It was a dream. It's all over.

The following days weigh you down like a ton of concrete. Everything is burdensome, meaningless. Every step is heavy. Your shoulders are drooping. Your muscles are tense, your gut is on strike. You are cold, all the way from your toes to your ears. Life is grey, as grey as your face. Until the miracle happens. Because you notice the tiny tear in your jacket. The ultimate secret hiding place. In your 'I've won the lottery' trance, you completely forgot about it. All of a sudden, you begin to glow. You begin to blossom.

Energy: *en* for 'internal', *ergon* for 'to operate'. One single piece of information can be enough to turn our entire system on its head. One thought can influence our entire physiology. And what are thoughts and information if not energy? They are devoid of material form, they cannot be physically grasped. They are flighty, non-tangible, unquantifiable. And yet no one would question their existence and the effect they can have. Our individual energy balance is, to a high degree, connected to our inner experiencing. TCM takes it a step further. It assumes that it is our internal energy that significantly shapes our external world, ranging from our body to all the manifestations with which we surround ourselves. Our consciousness determines our being. Just consider your life plan: isn't it the sum of all your ideas, your desires and the decisions you have made or didn't make? The nice house with a garden hasn't fallen into your lap, nor has the profession you took up. A well-toned body doesn't come about just like that, and nor does its opposite. Without exception, all objects in your environment, ranging from your computer to your car to your clothes, at some time in the past were no more than an idea that was then consistently implemented. Put differently: a large part of our life is nothing but energy that has become matter.

Meridians as Maps of the Soul

Now please stand up and walk over to the mirror. Look at your chin, your jawline, your lips. What do you see? Do you have the potential to bite through an iron bar? Or does a chewy slice of bread take you to your limits? How firmly can you 'bite' and do you show this? Is the lower third of your face wide and prominent? Do you have strong masticatory muscles? Do you have strong teeth ready to snap at something? Are you discovering the secret traits of a white shark within you? Yes? If you are male, congratulations! These facial features are generally rated as attractive, as masculine.

This is quite simply facial diagnosis according to TCM. What is evaluated here is the state of the stomach meridian. A strong stomach meridian results in a strong bite. And if you have a good bite, you can be as stubborn as a terrier with a bone, taking from the world what you need. You can be assertive and get your way, looking benevolently on the always richly laden smorgasbord of life. This is very inviting. It gives security and confidence. People who are able to provide for themselves are also able to provide for others. These qualities are generally considered attractive: an archaic appraisal. The power of our genes is certainly coming into play here: whether it's Brad Pitt, George Clooney or Leonardo di Caprio – open the multicoloured pages of your favourite magazine and you will notice that the alpha animals of our society all show the distinct features of a conspicuous stomach meridian. That's why they took their places at the head of the queue for the buffet of life. The same is true, of course, for female alpha animals like Madonna, Jennifer Lawrence or Hillary Clinton. The stomach meridian dominates their facial features, too. Meridians are like maps of the soul, expressing themselves on the landscape of the body.

But back to you standing in front of the mirror, back to your stomach meridian, your bite, your jaw. Of course, how your features are shaped partially depends on your genes and your parents. But what you have made of this inheritance is entirely down to you. Our inner energy forms our outer appearance. Even the strongest jaw can be drooping down listlessly when the appetite for life has been lost. And with sufficient tenacity, even a weak jaw can turn into a weapon of assertion, provided the hunger to achieve this is great enough. What you make of your disposition shows how strongly your stomach meridian is developed and how well you have integrated it. Our body is like a history book about our development. The meridians are a means to help us learn to read this book. And with our destiny in mind, we can learn to continue writing the story.

From Reading to Writing: What the Meridians Can Teach Us

We can consciously write and shape our life. What the meridians are asking us is this: have we integrated their respective life principles, and, if so, in what manner have we done this? The state of our musculature, our inner organs, our sensory organs and all our physiological functions allow us to recognise which strengths we have developed and where there are still challenges and tasks.

It does say something about us whether we approach life with sagging shoulders or with an upright posture, chest out and shoulders back. We embody our inner attitude through our external posture and our behaviour. Based on our stature, we position ourselves in life. The meridians, as maps of the soul, provide us with the map for a treasure hunt that allows us to discover and balance ourselves. Because balance is crucial.

Every person has strengths and every person has weaknesses.

That's completely normal. Remember the bicycle. If the wheel has only one strong spoke, it won't run smoothly for very long. The other spokes have to be at least strong enough to provide a sufficient counterbalance. It's the same with our strengths. Let's stay with the stomach meridian a little bit longer. In some people, it is overly conspicuous. They are very good at 'biting' their way through life and will go far. However, there is the danger that despite being so successful, they think they still don't have enough, that they have to keep doing more and more, all the way to burnout. In addition, such go-getters have a tendency to be extremely selfish, even narcissistic, so that the social aspects of their lives might suffer. Wealth on the outside, emotional emptiness inside. It takes a constructive balance for our strengths not to turn into weaknesses.

The meridian principle is based on twelve fundamental life principles. Each and every one of these principles requires development and integration in order to achieve the full potential of one's personality, to recognise and reach the truly important goals in life. This process could also be referred to as self-actualisation. Only through self-actualisation does our existence become meaningful. Every human being wants to grow and achieve their individual blossoming. Isn't that precisely why we have been born? True health is not the absence of illness. True health is growth on all levels.

Chapter 2

The Evolution of the Meridians

About Being Shipwrecked and Living on an Island: Maslow's Hierarchy of Needs

A long-held dream, finally fulfilled: the big crossing of the Pacific, in a sailing boat, as befits your standards. But then a storm, a hurricane, waves as high as a house, being shipwrecked, a lifebelt. You're drifting on the ocean; you're thirsty, hungry, tired, and there are only three things you really want: to survive, something to drink, to be saved. But fate treats you well, and you're washed up on a beach where, thank heavens, you find water and fruit. Otherwise, it's looking pretty bleak. You don't know where you are. You don't know how big the island is. You don't know anything, except that it would be wonderful to have shelter. You spend the next few days with a simple routine: foraging for food, sleeping, constructing something akin to a little house with branches and leaves, and, in between, hoping, again and again, to be rescued, for a miracle. At first, you were simply glad to have survived, but slowly the situation you're in is beginning to gnaw at your soul. All alone. On an island in the middle of nowhere. Maybe for ever...

Could that be possible? Perhaps! What if someone else had run ashore here, another victim of the foul weather? You're longing for company, a bit of human interaction. Being together instead of alone. A sorrow shared is a sorrow halved. Hope shared is hope doubled. You start searching, and at the other end of the island you make a discovery: another lost soul, another pitiful shelter. That's good. But how do you get together? It's what you make of a place that gives you a feeling of belonging, even if it is only a small emergency shelter. Who is willing to give up theirs? Who can offer more? You. Because you have a river next to your shack. That's your trump card; it makes things easier. Life goes on. And yet...what about being rescued? That's still uncertain. If it will happen at all. Days pass, weeks pass. In order not to go completely crazy, you begin to construct pieces of art out of driftwood on the beach, as big as possible. Perhaps someone will spot them. This keeps you occupied. It gives meaning to your existence. Because everybody has needs. The American psychologist Abraham Maslow categorised these.

The result is Maslow's pyramid of human needs, which assumes that our goals can be arranged in a hierarchical order. Oxygen and food are much more important than a Mercedes or a PhD. The base of the pyramid is therefore formed by our basic needs – that is, all the things a human being can't do without in order to survive. These include food, water, sleep, warmth and also reproduction. This is the first level that has to be secured.

Once the foundation is provided for, we can slowly begin to work on other little routines in order not to have to fight every day, again and again, for the things we need to live. Maslow refers to this second level as safety needs. They include safety and personal security, protection, as well as a place that provides a feeling of belonging. It's about material stability. Once this has been established, there will finally be time and space to devote oneself to interpersonal needs. Humans are, after all, social creatures. The third level therefore deals with belonging, friendship, family and love.

A full belly, a roof above your head and a little community – that's not bad at all. It's a good starting point for the vanity fair since every ego needs a little bit of balm. The fourth level addresses recognition, status, respect and power. It's about the need for individuation, about beginning to develop one's personality. The tip of the pyramid, the fifth level, stands for self-actualisation, for making the most of one's potential; for becoming a person who, based on their predisposition, has reached their full potential.

Maslow's model demonstrates that in different life situations we are motivated by different needs, as well as the importance of satisfying those needs. It doesn't have to be 100% satisfaction, but the relevant needs should be satisfied to a degree where it's possible to direct one's focus towards something else other than survival. In a nutshell: a hole in one's tummy isn't a motivation for self-development, and a hefty overdraft can get in the way of realising one's self. If we are desperately starving for love and recognition, we are less likely to be thirsting for realising bigger visions we have for our lives. What preoccupies us takes up our attention and energy. In order to reach the tip of the pyramid, we need the kit that is necessary to master the challenges of each level. To this end, the meridian system is an excellent source of help. After all, meridians, too, are governed by a certain hierarchy.

A Little Family Story: How Meridians Develop

At last, the longed-for baby is here. Barely arrived in this world, there is already much to do: sleeping, drinking, digesting, eliminating. But not everything goes smoothly from day one. While the sensitive digestive tract is developed, it has not fully matured yet. Certain intestinal bacteria are still missing, as are certain enzymes. Although drinking occurs instinctively, it is still somewhat uncoordinated. Sometimes a bit too much, sometimes not enough. And then there's the air that is swallowed along with the milk. The result: belching and bloating. It's time for burping and tummy massages. It's also time for patience: it can take months until the guts and everything else have got used to their new tasks and work as a well-practised team. The lungs, in contrast, had to learn much faster, being fully required as soon as the umbilical cord was cut. The vital first breath would have initiated a cascade of processes playing a central role for the entire organism. It's the lungs that allow the big jump into independent life. It's the same in Traditional Chinese Medicine, since the evolution of the meridians has a direct connection to our human development. Traditional Chinese Medicine views these processes in exactly the same way, because the evolution of the meridians has a direct connection to our development as humans.

In an infant, the meridians involved with respiration, digestion and elimination are particularly active. Just as the little organism is learning and evolving, the meridians learn and evolve, too. They grow alongside the body. They determine growth as there is a direct interaction between information and matter. Meridians are like an energetic code, manifesting the life principle they represent in all levels of our body. Conversely, the body's development shapes the coding of the meridians, step by step, according to the developmental phase. And each phase has a particular focus. Survival has to be safeguarded first, requiring the organism to be supplied with oxygen and energy. Then there is the elimination of waste products and protection against illness. All these functions are covered by the tasks of the meridians pertaining to the lung, stomach, large intestine and spleen respectively.

The meridian system comprises twelve main meridians which can be grouped in various ways. Best known is the system of the Five Elements, which lends itself beautifully to describing pathological processes affecting the organs. For the representation of childhood developmental processes, the meridians are arranged to form meridian families, with four meridians forming a unit that fulfils a supraordinate communal task. This task reflects the most important learning steps of a human's developmental process. Within its group, each meridian contributes to the requirements of the relevant task by virtue of its specific embodied life principle. Twelve meridians are divided into three meridian families with four meridians each. Twelve meridians thus represent three big developmental chapters and twelve fundamental life principles.

The first meridian family deals with the questions: Am I able to provide for myself? Am I able to feed myself? It refers to all levels of human existence – material, emotional, mental – and also corresponds to the first three levels of Maslow's hierarchy of needs.

The core questions of the second meridian family are: Who am I? What do I want? This family is represented by the meridians of the heart, small intestine, bladder and kidney. These meridians begin to develop when the infant learns to move, to articulate itself; when the child discovers its 'I' and its will. The second meridian family has a connection with the fourth level of Maslow's pyramid, concerned with individual needs.

When we are able to care for ourselves, when we know who we are and what we want, the next step is to express this in the form of a vision that activates our full potential. This self-actualisation is the task of the third meridian family, the final one to develop, forming the tip of Maslow's pyramid of needs. The meridians of the pericardium, liver, triple heater and gallbladder provide vigour, passion and coordination, and the ability to plan.

With the meridians developing well, this brings us back to the wheel, with all its spokes finely aligned and correctly tightened. Everything is running smoothly. You're rolling nonchalantly and easily through life, towards your destiny. That would be the ideal scenario. But not every road has an even surface. Often there are potholes and stones that cause us to wobble, especially on the road of our personal development.

The Leaning Tower of Pisa: About the Dents in Our Life Story

The Leaning Tower of Pisa is famous for its very obvious tilt. The root of the problem is the substrate, a mix of loamy swamp and sand. Not the best base on which to construct a massive building. But people weren't deterred. It took 200 years in total to complete the structure, and who knows if the tower would still be standing if it had not been for repeated comprehensive restorations. What the Leaning Tower of Pisa teaches us is that it all depends on the foundations. But what has this to do with the meridian principle?

Let's look at the newborn baby again. Let's assume the infant is optimally cared for: milk, regular nappy changes, a comfortable temperature, a mechanically induced simulation of movement, everything perfect. But...no body contact, no cuddles, no social interaction – nothing. It is as if you were putting a plant into soil but depriving it of the sun. This plant would not grow well; it would probably wither. It has been scientifically proven that the same happens with children. Growing is not just about satisfying needs on a functional level. It's also about soul food. It requires affection and emotional warmth as well as a heartfelt welcome towards the entire being.

Without warmth and affection, it would be difficult, even impossible, to build any form of trust. Insecurity and fear, in turn, are bad fertilisers for personal growth. They result in massive dents in the developmental wheel, which make it difficult to satisfactorily pursue certain needs, such as the need for closeness and relationships. Or there may be a permanent deficiency: the feeling of being unloved, of not being accepted. A foundation riddled with insecurity about emotional relationships can lead to instability affecting the entire structure. Just as with the Leaning Tower of Pisa.

In principle, every meridian can develop a dent at any time. Even the most solid foundation can be shaken by an earthquake. Either way, it's much harder to move forward when the developmental wheel is dented. Sometimes we may even come to a complete standstill, pedalling on the spot. Life won't be running smoothly then. In fact, it won't be running at all.

How the Meridians and Their Life Principles Gain Strength

A poorly developed, unintegrated life principle is like a weak point that can affect our entire life, until we take active steps to deal with it. We can let every life principle unfold anew, even if it is barely present. We can strengthen the development of every meridian. We only have to find out what it takes to strengthen the affected spokes in the wheel of our life.

Each meridian is presented in a separate chapter. These chapters describe in great detail the life principle embodied by the respective meridians and how this is expressed in our bodies. In this context, the connection between body, mind and emotions takes centre stage. Acupuncture points can be seen as a particularly concentrated expression of the relevant meridian energy and its associated life principle. For this reason, the most important acupuncture points have also been included, along with references to their functions and what they communicate.

Questions and exercises for promoting the life principles of the meridians provide an opportunity for self-reflection. For those who haven't had much exposure to TCM and the meridians, this will be exciting new territory. It is my hope that therapists of a wide range of backgrounds will find this book helpful in adding to their knowledge and deepening their work.

PART II

THE LIFE PRINCIPLES OF THE MERIDIANS

Introduction to Part II

The meridians are arranged according to the organ clock, which symbolises the order in which the meridians develop and evolve in our body. While each meridian embodies a fundamental life principle, they have many further functions that are either linked to or support their core function. Although a clear focus emerges for each meridian, the qualities of many meridians are similar or overlap. Some meridians have a protective function, some have to do with opening up our body, others facilitate balance and harmony. This is due to the fact that meridians interact and complement each other when it comes to the bigger picture. In addition, meridians are coupled with each other. Each meridian is assigned to one of the Five Elements. Each element is associated with one yin and one yang meridian, except for the fire element, which is allocated two yin and two yang meridians. The meridians pertaining to the same element are referred to as partnered meridians; they form a pair that belongs together. They tend to shed light on the same subject, albeit it from two different angles.

Then there are the twinned meridians, which are similar in the way they relate to the physical structure of the body. For example, the lung meridian courses along the inside of the arm, and the spleen meridian along the inside of the leg. They influence similar areas of the body – in this case, the medial aspects of the limbs – yet they focus on different core themes, just as the arms and legs can be grouped together as extremities despite having different functions. The tasks of twinned meridians can also display similarities and overlaps.

Some meridians may have a stronger connection to the body, others are more closely related to emotions, and yet others to our mind and consciousness. For this reason, the weighting of their principal aspects isn't always the same. Some meridians are associated with a host of physical pathologies, while others are more prone to mental and emotional problems.

The best starting point is to read the questions for the meridians at the beginning of each chapter. If that touches you emotionally or you feel a little bit caught out, engaging with that particular meridian could turn into an exciting journey for you! Enjoy!

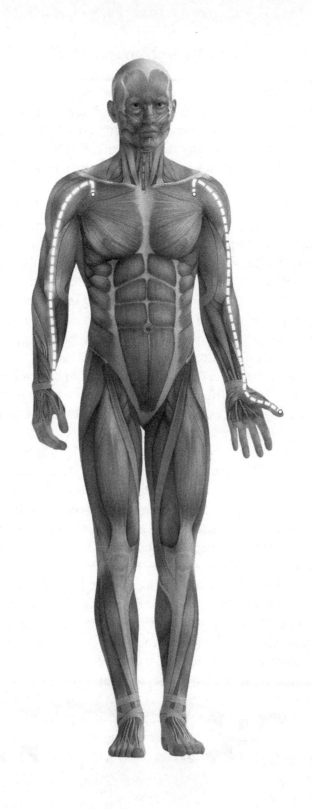

Chapter 3

The Lung Meridian

The Big 'Yes' to Life

Questions for the Lung Meridian

- Am I able to say 'yes' loudly and clearly?
- Do I have a positive view of myself and my future?
- Do I find it easy to be open to new things?
- Do I take up the space that I am due?
- Do I observe and respect boundaries?
- Do I have sufficient vitality and strength?
- Do I tend to rely on my instincts?

The Life Principle of the Lung Meridian

In the organ clock according to TCM, the lungs take first place. They start the energy circulation of the meridians. It is the lungs that make the river of life flow. It is with the lungs and a feisty yawn that we greet each awakening day. It is with the lungs and a deep breath that we endeavour to take new steps or make important decisions. And, above all, it's with the lungs that we begin our independent journey as human beings. Taking our first breath after the umbilical cord has been cut, we connect with a completely different world. After months of coming into being and maturing in a protective and consistent environment, we encounter the outer world for the very first time. We open up. We allow the external world to pour into us. The first breath is very special: it activates a cascade of reactions that are crucial for the body of the newborn child. Without this breath, there would be no leap into one's own existence. Without the first big 'yes' to survival, there would be no beginning. Saying 'yes' is the power of the lung meridian.

Each 'yes' is like a door that we open with affirming goodwill and benevolence in order to let in new things. A well-developed lung meridian radiates confidence and accessibility. It responds to the future and what is unknown with a positive attitude. It is a dynamic optimist: whatever may come, a strong lung will say 'yes' because it can rely on its long, energising breath. With a long and steady breath, obstacles can be overcome and boundaries moved. Saying 'yes' means not giving up. It means persevering, keeping going. Saying 'yes' means being constructively connected to the river of life. This creates a tail wind and a good mood.

If, on the other hand, the life principle of the lung meridian is only poorly developed, matters can deflate pretty quickly. Even small things take our breath away, unforeseen events leave us holding our breath, changes tighten our chest, and it doesn't take much for our shoulders to droop. Therefore, and purely as a precaution, there's no 'yes' to the future but rather a loud and clear 'maybe' to every small step. After all, who knows what will be? Surely nothing good. While this assumption is obviously as wrong as 'all will be well', it has a completely different feel to it – and also different consequences. It can cause a promising beginning to come to a sudden halt, quite simply because it doesn't give space to any potential possibility, but rather slams the door shut right in its face. A 'yes' opens and is a beginning; a 'no' closes and terminates. The most profound 'no' we will ever experience occurs with our last breath – the final exhalation. We end our journey on planet earth the same way we started it – with our lungs.

The life principle of the lung meridian stands not only for an unshakeable affirmation of life; it also stands for saying 'yes' to oneself, for a healthy connection with the self. Strong lung energy allows us to accept ourselves the way we are, and it allows us to take and to grant ourselves precisely the amount of space adequate for our needs and goals at a particular time, so that we always have sufficient air to keep breathing. The life principle of the lungs helps us to develop a healthy egoism, ensuring that we always hold our head high to where the air is fresh and invigorating, rather than fighting for the leftovers of life's buffet in the musty depths of everyday trivialities.

Saying 'yes' to ourselves also manifests in an extremely robust constitution. Strong lung energy results in a powerful body, in overflowing vitality, in a strong immune system. A wide chest that is filled to the brim. It's for a reason that the chest is also where the lung meridian begins. It provides people with a proud and self-confident demeanour. Add to this a thick skin that is able to endure and tolerate a lot. In TCM, the skin is associated with the lungs since it, too, breathes, opens and closes. The skin can act as a well-functioning shield, a clear boundary. Thus forearmed, it takes a lot to ruffle someone's feathers: one feels happy and content in one's skin.

With all these conditions fulfilled, it is easy to open up to life and relate well to other people. A lung meridian with a strong life principle is the foundation for openness and communication. It allows people to be daring. It gives them a can-do attitude and the will to follow things through. Being touched is experienced as enjoyable, as is touching others. It's about being both permeable and resilient.

A disharmony of the lung meridian's life principle, however, is a completely different story. In such a case, the forever hopeful and cheerful 'yes' can quickly turn into a vehement 'no'. People say 'no' to themselves, 'no' to life, 'no' to getting up in the morning, 'no' to the coming day, 'no' to any possibility, 'no' to the past, 'no' to the present. The in-breath is full of negativity, and thus toxic. This can lead to a deep denial of one's personality, to self-sabotage, to self-destructive thinking and acting, and, in extreme cases, to a lingering pessimism and even a refusal to live. And on top of all that, such people tend to have a very thin skin, making them terribly sensitive and vulnerable. They feel everything intensely; everything touches them deeply, but defence is impossible because their 'no' also has an effect on their physical strength, which is in the doldrums. In other words, people feel as though they want to crawl out of their skin.

The only thing that can help is to stay calm, breathe deeply and, step by step, reclaim the 'yes' to life. A life-affirming and also self-affirming attitude of the lung meridian is the life principle on which those of all other meridians are based. Because there cannot be a beginning without a 'yes'.

The Lung Meridian and the Body

Mountain Gorillas, Elves and Breathing

The lungs are our primary energy source. We can manage without food for quite some time. Without drink, things get tight much more quickly. But without breathing, alarm bells go off straight away. The expansion and contraction of the lungs form the rhythm of our breathing. The lungs ensure that carbon dioxide, a waste product of metabolic processes, is exhaled and replaced by fresh oxygen. Fresh oxygen is life; it is vitality. Inhaling is saying 'yes' to something new; exhaling is getting rid of what no longer serves us. If this rhythm stagnates, the old remains within us, and the new can't enter. There is no longer any exchange, no interaction between the interior and exterior. We sever the connection to life – with the corresponding consequences: it gets stuffy, as in a room that is never aired. We are polluted internally and become turbid, like water lacking oxygen. We get tired, devoid of drive, and lose all hope.

It is a particular trait of the lung meridian to compensate for this internal stagnation and pollution by exaggerated external cleanliness, including obsessive hygiene, pathological tidiness and excessive cleaning habits. These are an attempt at externally achieving the conditions – a neat and tidy environment – that are lacking internally. Each speck of dust is a source of resentment and declared a personal foe as it serves as a reminder of the internal build-up of increasing amounts of dirt caused by the insufficient exchange of air and the lack of a fresh breeze brought in by the breath. Separated from the pulsating river of the outside world, there is no inner cleansing or renewal. People try to compensate for this lack with three showers a day, by washing their hands umpteen times, accumulating an entire arsenal of deodorants and other personal care products, as well as having a clinically sterile home.

44

But the opposite can happen as well. Weak lung energy can lead to resignation and helplessness setting in. There is a state of deflation; there are hanging shoulders. There is never a 'yes' to anything, not even to the most basic self-care and care for one's immediate environment; rather, there is a yielding to decay and increasing neglect. Neither the body nor the clothing nor the dwelling place show any traces of freshness or vitality; it's all like a muddy pond full of decomposing matter. There is gradual pollution on all levels, which may go unnoticed as weak lung energy also affects the sense of smell. But regardless of whether there is excessive or inadequate care, both disharmonies can be a fertile breeding ground for skin problems and allergies as the protective shield becomes weakened. There is a disturbed relationship to the outside world, resulting in maladjusted reactions.

The external environment reflects the state of the lung energy, and not just regarding hygiene. The respiratory volume of the lungs is determined by many factors but the key that facilitates taking a truly deep breath can often be found in the mind. The crucial questions for the lung meridian are therefore: How much space do I grant myself? Do I have the courage to expand my potential and my needs, both internally and externally? Am I breathing powerfully and vigorously? Do I make full use of the respiratory volume available to me? Do I make full use of the space that is my due? Do I go all the way to its limits? Or is my breathing shallow and far below my capacity? Am I constricting myself and tightening my own chest? Is the way I live as shallow as the way I breathe?

TCM considers the lungs the architect of the body. Good lung energy manifests in a powerful physical presence, a robust constitution, along with strength, resilience and good health – a bit like King Kong, tending towards invincibility. Each pore oozes vitality. Energy levels are high. At the other end of the spectrum are the elves: an ethereal aura, a weak chest, highly sensitive, often tired as well as despondent, with a tendency towards porcelain skin and feeling overwhelmed by life. In summary, a fragile appearance lacking stability and assertiveness should the wind of life turn into a gale as it sometimes does. The life principle of the lungs is mirrored in the architect's mindset. A strong 'yes' to life will create strong buildings. An uncertain 'no', on the other hand, will render the entire construction unstable, since both planning and execution are hampered by much insecurity and a lack of stable breathing needed for good stamina.

But it's not just about the quality of the building, it's also about how the building is lived in. Our respiration is the bridge between our psyche and our physical body. Whether we choose meditation, self-hypnosis or modern stress management, we know that deep, relaxed breathing can unite the head and the body to form one constructive unit. Once this connection has been established, we will feel content and at home in our body. This creates a feeling of self-awareness and security, just as with the King Kong type. He doesn't question his identity. His ego is as healthy and stable as his material shell. The 'yes' to himself is loud and clear. He gets what he needs; he takes up his space, if required, with forceful assertion – classic territorial behaviour. On a physical level, we find instinctive responses, which are typical of people with strong lung energy. They are endowed with a well-developed sixth sense. They can sense danger, smell worthwhile opportunities and react quickly. Their home is in the jungle of life, and they like to take up a big territory.

It's much harder for the elves. With elves, you never know whether they have actually landed on this planet or whether they are still floating somewhere in the sky. Their 'yes' to life is replaced by a huge question mark: What on earth am I doing here? Am I supposed to be on this planet, or should I be somewhere else? Why do I have this body and what am I supposed to do with it? Their physical presence is more like some form of abstinence. They breathe so delicately and quietly that you can never be sure whether they are breathing at all. Or you worry that they may simply dissolve and vanish into thin air. The lungs, in their capacity as architect, have constructed a fragile building that requires to be handled with care. Reaction patterns, instincts, immunity as well as the 'yes' to the self are only poorly developed. They take up little internal and external space, boundaries turn into grey areas – does there remain anything at all of the self?

In both cases, it can be helpful to consider the life principle of the lung meridian. If it's too strong, the result will be a form of egoism that doesn't leave much space for anyone else. And if it's too weak, people constantly leave their personal space to others. A happy medium would be the ability for self-care and occupying one's space in life while keeping it open and inviting for others.

Allergies (in particular, dust, animal hair, pollen), chronic fatigue, chronically weak immune system, susceptible to frequent infections, shortness of breath, chest tightness, fear of confined or open spaces, asthma, weak constitution, poor instincts, impaired reaction patterns...

Feeling Content in One's Skin

In TCM, the skin, as our largest respiratory organ, belongs to the organ system of the lungs and has an important function, both physically and psychologically. It represents the interface between inner and outer space, between the internal and external world. The skin facilitates contact and exchange. Ideally, it will be elastic, permeable and resistant. The skin mirrors how well the lungs' life principle was able to evolve in our body. Once again, the body's architect comes into play here: What kind of barrier have they constructed around the building? A thick wall that provides good protection but is impermeable? Or just a few rickety planks which will collapse simply by being looked at? Do we have a thick or a thin skin? Is there really nothing that gets our hackles up, or do we instantly have an allergic reaction?

A thick skin is like a carapace. The hatches are battened down. The door is closed. The pores are sealed. It's difficult to truly touch someone like that because everything will bounce back off the protective layer encasing their core, both the good and also the less good things in life, but especially feelings. And it's precisely feelings that thick-skinned people prefer to avoid; they don't want to 'feel'. Nothing is let in, nothing is taken personally, nothings gets under their skin. People like that appear aloof and distant, but ultimately they are trapped within themselves. They become rigid as if they were wearing a rusty suit of armour. Once again, what's lacking is a healthy exchange with the outside world so much appreciated by the lung meridian. This is a kind of stagnation that makes people want to crawl out of their skin, but they're so stuck in it that it's completely impossible. Sooner or later, any stagnation results in a build-up of pressure, and, over time, pressure results in heat. People begin to burn internally, which is expressed through acne or atopic dermatitis. The internal blaze tries to open up a pathway, as in a volcano. It's bubbling under the surface, and now and again some lava is spluttering to the outside, clearly visible in the red craters on the skin. Otherwise there's nothing much to see. Even the sweat finds it hard to penetrate the surface towards the outside. This is an attempt to prevent others picking up the scent and getting a whiff of how someone is doing. According to TCM, the sweat, being a clear liquid, may congeal, and the skin may become greasy, the result being sebaceous deposits. Frequently, this results in a colourful rash – and it's clearly visible from afar. This is not a healthy state of affairs.

It's not any easier for very thin-skinned people. They take everything personally, as if they were running the gauntlet without any recourse to resources. Any kind of triviality is sufficient to make them feel under attack. They react with slight irritation, get nervous quickly, start to sweat; the pores open up, and everything can get in, everything can get out. It's difficult to hide anything; the skin doesn't provide any protection. They feel literally skinned, naked down to the flesh. This hypersensitivity results in the feeling that they constantly have to defend their skin since they are missing natural boundaries and the healthy protective function of their skin. The resulting strategy is withdrawal and isolation, accompanied by the attempt to become invisible in order to avoid any confrontation. This, too, can be at the bottom of skin problems – for example, in contact allergies, which can act as a warning: 'Keep your distance! Don't touch me! I am already very irritated!' Sometimes even natural sunlight can be too much. The slightest stimulus can result in burning. There will be a tendency to sensitive, chapped skin that easily becomes inflamed. Such people can also be prone to dandruff or scaly skin, like scales falling off the faulty armour. And because everything is a source of irritation, there is often itching. Or urticaria, since everything is prickly. Regardless of whether it's thick or thin, who wants skin like that?

But what can you do to feel happy in your skin? Regularly shed your skin, leaving the tightening shell behind. Growth is like saying 'yes' to life, 'yes' to one's self. It strengthens the life principle of the lungs. People who have a good relationship with their environment, and who are confident to open up when appropriate and to close when necessary, are considered honest souls. People like that make you feel that 'what you see is what you get' – and what you see is the surface, the skin. This conscious opening and closing is something that needs to be learned.

SYMPTOMS ASSOCIATED WITH THE LUNG MERIDIAN

Dry skin, skin that is easily chapped, easily inflamed skin, dandruff, oily skin, too much or too little sweating, acne, atopic dermatitis, psoriasis, contact allergies, sun allergy, itching, urticaria...

The Lung Meridian and the Psyche

Past, Present and Future

Breathing plays a key role in all meditation techniques. By focussing on the breath, we're neither in the past nor in the future. We are in the here and now – the only place in time and space where we can live and experience life. But it's not easy to get there just like that. Our thoughts like to jump about, hither and thither. They skip to what could be or to what was. By concentrating on the breath, we connect our awareness with our body. And our body can be nowhere else but in precisely this spot in precisely this moment. This is the principle of meditation.

If there is one spot our thoughts tend to jump to, it's backwards, to those events that have led to the droopy shoulders and the shortness of breath. But that's also the spot where our future-loving lungs suffer the most. In TCM, grief is the emotion with the greatest influence on the lungs. Grief is the normal reaction to loss, and grieving requires time: what has happened needs to be processed, wounds have to heal. A further part of this process is the gradual letting go of the emotional and mental links with the relevant event. If the lungs' life principle is well developed, it will have the capacity to achieve that. It has the capacity to grieve well. But an imbalanced lung meridian will struggle; it will look back rather than ahead. It will constantly drag a part of our consciousness to the past, mourning for the good old days. When we are fearful of the future, it's easier to live with past experiences. Or we find it difficult to cope with loss and to make a new beginning. Our grief is never fully processed, never fully concluded. There may be grieving for a lost person, missed opportunities, wasted time. For the lungs' energy, this is as if we had inhaled and were holding our breath. We preserve the used air instead of opening up to new horizons, thus forgoing new perspectives and opportunities. We turn into a sad person, and sad people tend to adopt a rather pessimistic outlook on life.

Having strong lungs is like having wings. In a weak lung meridian, the wings are clipped, so much so that there's no point in even thinking about flying. But that's something that people with an imbalanced lung meridian dislike anyway, because they're convinced from the outset that flying at high altitudes will ultimately end in a crash. They are not only scared that their actions will fail to bring the desired results, but they anticipate the worst. Even with the most colourful crayons, they produce only black pictures – in their eyes, that's the only colour the future holds. They are born pessimists. Theirs is a vicious cycle requiring urgent disruption to prevent the descent into a chronically depressed state.

Therefore: please shed your entire skin and let yourself be born anew. A healthy, well-developed lung energy always has the strength for a new beginning. In this endeavour, our respiration is crucial. Our breath can liberate us from the grasp of the past and allow us to return to the present moment. And if this moment connects with the life-affirming power of the lung energy, it can bring us back to the future. Lungs with a strong life principle are the foundation of an unshakeable yet realistic optimism. It is the insight that optimism will bring to a positive outlook that turbo-charges our vitality and courage. People with strong lung energy always look at the glass half-full anyway, pondering how to make it even fuller. They have plans. They have a long, powerful breath providing them with a constant tail wind. Impending obstacles don't rob them of their air. They don't interpret a backlash as a harbinger of failure but rather as a learning curve on the path to their goal, allowing them to sustain a positive spirit and vigour. They cultivate a solution-oriented attitude and strive to fulfil their potential because they believe in the future – their future.

Contact, Boundaries and Communication

The lungs are the only organ that has a direct contact and connection with the outside world. Our respiration – and also our skin – facilitates a continuous exchange with our environment. But not just the lungs; each system in our body, each cell, requires such an exchange in order to survive, to regenerate and to maintain vitality. To this end, each system and each cell has to be discernible as a discrete entity, and this requires boundaries defining such cohesive units. A cell without a membrane will dissolve. A river without a riverbed that contains it will dissolve. A house without walls, a roof or at least some minimal structure is no house. And a person without boundaries finds it very hard to develop an awareness of themselves and others. Boundaries provide clarity. This is my space. That is your space. I am here. You are there. Only with clear boundaries can there be conscious contact and, subsequently, a conscious exchange between people.

Contact and exchange with our environment are important aspects of the life principle of the lung meridian. Contact and exchange are the essential building blocks of communication between humans; they are indispensable for our personal growth and health. Social isolation can indeed cause illness, ranging from lowered immunity to an increased risk of Alzheimer's disease. Humans need humans. We share emotions, thoughts, opinions and information with others to self-validate and learn. Just as the breath exchanges stale air for fresh, the exchange facilitated through communication can lead to a new impetus and outlook, which can contribute to letting go of habits or views that no longer serve us. Communication is a process facilitating change and growth. But any constructive interaction also involves listening and taking in. The lung meridian takes care of this.

There are two ways in which an imbalanced life principle of the lungs can manifest. Some people attempt to take up a great deal of space in the way they communicate. They talk loudly and brashly. Empty phrases serve for both attack and defence. Communication turns into a one-way street to the exclusion of oncoming traffic. Contact serves as an ego boost, not as an exchange. Without any true connection, the conversation can be about one person only: oneself. Exaggerated self-centredness, associated with imbalances of the lung meridian, shows its ugly face. Others are interrupted, and one's topic is pursued at all costs. This form of communication separates. One talks a lot, and yet one is alone.

If, however, the boundaries are too weak, a person will constantly adapt to the people around them; everything is taken in, and it's taken personally. A grey zone arises, in which one's own position is not clearly recognisable. Identities become blurred. It's easier to acquiesce, easier to say 'yes' to everything, easier to simply listen rather than contribute something. This makes it almost impossible to establish a conscious, meaningful connection, since such a person is not really present in the conversation. It further leads to avoidance or even fear of contact. In a nutshell: some people like to influence, while others like to be influenced. However, this is of no benefit for either party since contact is such important nourishment for the soul. We need healthy interaction in order to stay healthy.

If the lungs' life principle is well developed, there will be clear boundaries allowing a conscious exchange. We will say 'yes' to ourselves and 'yes' to others. We will be aware that, similarly to the breath, growth and further personal development can only arise through a continuous exchange.

Signs of an Imbalanced and Balanced Lung Meridian

Signs of an Imbalanced Lung Meridian

- Delicate constitution, reduced vitality, poor immunity
- Susceptible to frequent colds and flu, fatigue, lack of motivation
- Depressed demeanour, deflated, fear of the future

- Poor boundaries, everything is taken personally
- Pronounced egoism, overstepping the boundaries of others, aloof
- Difficulty with genuine opening up and true contact
- Poor intuition and weak reaction patterns

Signs of a Balanced Lung Meridian

- Robust build, strong vitality, good immunity
- Optimistic and life-affirming attitude
- Perseverance, patience and tenacity
- Good sense of personal boundaries and also those of others, good spatial perception
- Excellent intuition, sixth sense, quick reaction patterns
- Conscious opening and closing, good rapport with people

How to Strengthen the Life Principle of the Lung Meridian

Beginning the Day with an Affirmative 'Yes'

Early morning is the time of the lungs. Set your alarm 15 minutes earlier than your normal getting-up time. As you wake, turn to lie on your back, place one hand on your chest, the other on your belly, and deepen your breathing so that a calm and strong rhythm arises. Then ask yourself the following questions: What am I looking forward to today? What good things could happen to me today? What would I like to achieve today? Try to let any arising images be as realistic as possible, closing each visualisation with an optimistic 'yes' to yourself. Develop a joyful anticipation and curiosity for the day ahead.

And then it's all go: Yes! Get yourself what you need to let those images become reality, even if it requires a bit more egoism. You're not acting egoistically because you want to boost your self-worth. You're acting egoistically because you want to care for yourself well and with a positive attitude. Treat yourself to the space that is genuinely yours. Don't make yourself little. Make yourself big. Make yourself even bigger. Don't accept any compromise. Again, and again, take a deep breath and say loudly and clearly 'yes' to yourself.

Boost the Fighting Spirit

The lungs really like a physical challenge: walk as far as you can and then again twice that distance. Play-fight with someone much stronger than you are. Spend a whole day outdoors during extreme weather conditions. Willpower is good. Our will for survival is so strong since it is anchored at the deeper levels of our existence. It's connected to our survival instinct, which played such an important role when we took our first breath after birth. If you would like to strengthen the life principle of the lungs, then it is of great benefit if the 'yes' to life and survival is roused not only in the head but in each and every cell. This will only happen when we think we've gone as far as we can, when we're scratching at the limit and still go beyond. This approach will quickly and directly strengthen the life principle of the lungs.

The Pathway of the Lung Meridian

The pathway of the lung meridian begins below the collarbone, in the first intercostal space, six thumb-widths lateral to the midline, where we find Lung 1. From Lung 1, the meridian courses upward to Lung 2, located directly below the collarbone. The pathway continues along the collarbone towards the shoulder and along the anterior border of the deltoid, approximately a thumb-width superior to a horizontal groove formed by the deltoid and the large chest muscle (pectoralis major).

On the upper arm, the lung meridian follows the lateral aspect of the biceps. The next important landmark is Lung 5, located in the elbow crease, slightly lateral to the midline, on the inside border of the brachioradialis. From Lung 5, the lung meridian continues to follow the brachioradialis, initially on its muscle belly, then along its tendon. The straight line of the meridian is only broken by the point Lung 7, which can be found proximal to the styloid process at the distal end of the radius.

An important landmark on the wrist is Lung 9, located on the thumb-side of the wrist crease. Onwards from Lung 9, the lung meridian follows the bulky musculature at the base of the thumb (thenar eminence), close to the first metacarpal bone, and ends at the medial corner of the thumbnail at Lung 11.

Key Areas of the Lung Meridian

Chest and Shoulders

The pathway of the lung meridian begins in the chest – and for a good reason. The chest is an area where it will be most evident whether someone feels deflated, whether their shoulders are tiredly hanging downwards and whether they have a weak chest. Or whether someone walks through life with a puffed-out chest and sufficient strength to take on the world. The first point on the lung meridian is Lung 1, *zhong fu*, 'Middle Palace' or 'Middle Treasury'. Lung 1 is also the alarm point of the lung meridian. Alarm points have a direct connection to the overall energetic state of a meridian; accordingly, any conspicuous signs at such points indicate a state of alarm. But what is it that resides in this treasure house around Lung 1? It's our vitality, the strength of the life principle of the lungs. If the chest is weak and deficient, the lung meridian needs support, energy, space and oxygen. Otherwise, we'd collapse like a burst balloon. What is required is inhaling deeply, strengthening the 'yes' to life, a good supply of life force – in other words, generally filling up. Conversely, an excessively inflated balloon can easily burst, just like an inflated ego is prone to quickly explode. Lung 1 can therefore be not only too empty but also too full and puffed up. This calls for a good exhalation and permeability. Lung 1 is excellent for regulating either condition.

If there is sufficient energy and vitality, then it becomes much easier to open up and gaze at the horizon, towards what could lie ahead of us. An upright posture, positive curiosity – all this is expressed by Lung 2, the 'Cloud Gate' or *yun men*. Instead of pessimistically staring at the ground, we open the door to heaven.

Wrist and Thumbs

The strength of the wrists is a good indicator of whether the lungs, as architects of the body, have erected a robust or a flimsy building. At the wrists, we find another important point on the lung meridian, Lung 9, *tai yuan*, 'Deep Spring' or 'Supreme Abyss'. Being connected and having contact are major qualities of the lungs. If we are in contact with the 'deep spring' – that is, with ourselves and our environment – then we are not at the edge of a 'supreme abyss', threatened by isolation, life-negating attitudes and grief, and in danger of tumbling down. Lung 9 is also the area where we take the pulse. How much life energy is flowing through our body? Having little energy can throw us down into the abyss as we are too tired or exhausted to have the will to participate in life.

Our thumbs express our overall constitution. Thumbs-up means okay, everything's fine, all is well. Thumbs-down tells us 'no', we can't continue like this. The muscle belly at the base of the thumb, the thenar eminence, reflects the strength of our 'okay'. There we also find the point Lung 10, 'Fish Border' or *yu ji*, which derives its name from this area resembling a fish belly. Is this fish belly strong and powerful? Or is it looking sunken and flaccid? Lung 10 indicates how much joy and enthusiasm we find in the lung meridian. Lung 10 is the fire point of this meridian. Its message: a thumbs-up to life is better than sitting at home and twiddling your thumbs.

The Lung Meridian: Key Points

- Associated element: Metal element
- Quality: Yin
- Time on the organ clock: 3am–5am
- Animal quality: Tiger
- Partner meridian: Large intestine meridian
- Twinned meridian: Spleen meridian
- Opposite meridian: Bladder meridian

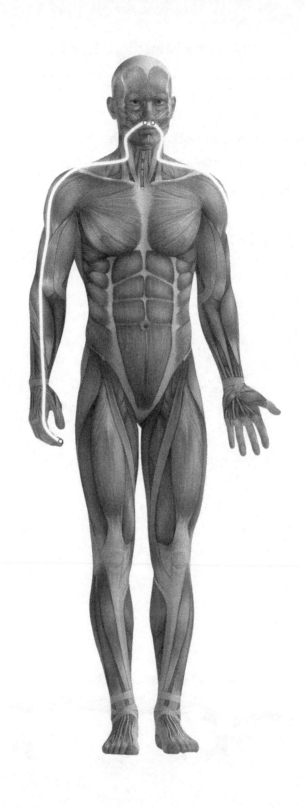

Chapter 4

The Large Intestine Meridian

The Power of 'No'

Questions for the Large Intestine Meridian

- Am I able to say 'no' loudly and clearly?
- Am I able to set boundaries and defend them?
- Am I able to control myself and my environment?
- Am I able to stick to something and persevere with it?
- Am I able to let go and relax?
- Am I able to put past events behind me and let go of them?
- Do I find it easy to relate to and deal with material matters?
- Do I easily feel guilty and try to acquiesce?

The Life Principle of the Large Intestine Meridian

In the beginning, everything ends up in a baby's nappies. Life is in a constant flow. And little baby flows along, too – instinctively, impetuously. It is only once the life principle of the large intestine meridian begins to develop that there is more control, mainly the consciously learned control of the anal sphincter. This is not easy, it takes time, but it is an important step towards self-control. At some point, the growing 'I' will have taken things into its own hands and is therefore able to consciously stop, postpone or let go of the flow of life passing through. Now the 'I' decides when and where it needs the potty. The large intestine meridian controls it all. This is its job and its mission. Above all, it likes to control through the power of 'no'.

Saying 'no' means to set boundaries. Saying 'no' means 'I don't want this!' Saying 'no' means 'This is not for me!' In our everyday life, we need the life principle of the large intestine meridian a lot. Without the ability to demarcate our territory with a conscious 'no', it is difficult to assert ourselves and our needs in challenging situations because we tend to say 'yes' all too quickly and too easily to anything and everything. We do this because we don't want to disappoint others, because we instantly feel guilty, because we are afraid not to be accepted or liked, because we have learned to be obedient. Because we prefer to clench our mental buttocks and suppress our needs and our views rather than get out the sword of resistance and risk a conflict. The sword of body language is the raised index finger. It warns. It admonishes. The raised index finger says 'no' and keeps things at a distance. And it's at the index finger where the pathway of the large intestine meridian begins.

A poorly developed life principle of the large intestine gives other people the opportunity to assert themselves and, without much effort, occupy any undefended space with their wishes, demands, opinions and emotions. And if they are not bidden farewell straight away, they will build their cosy nest in the basement of our consciousness. Without a clear 'no' acting as the gatekeeper, it will become quite crowded in our house as time goes on. It will get crammed and clogged. It's like constipation – in the heart, in one's life and, of course, in the large intestine. Or there may be diarrhoea, because all and sundry are marching through, as there is no one to put up any opposition. This requires energy and is tiring. Either way, eventually you find yourself up shit creek because you're constantly being dumped on. You'll be buried under a plethora of big brown piles which have nothing whatsoever to do with you, yet they grow bigger day by day. It's enough. It stinks to high heaven. You're completely fed up. Your nose can't bear the smell any longer. And that's where the large intestine meridian terminates – at the nose.

An imbalance of the large intestine meridian can lead to accumulations, and not only in the form of withheld stools or stuck waste products in the intestinal loops. Long-standing residual waste accumulates on all levels. This waste is a strain – in the short, medium and long term. A healthy large intestine meridian, on the other hand, finds it easy to dispose of the dung heaps that have become obsolete and no longer serve the body. It eliminates what is no longer of value. It says 'no' to the residual waste of the physical, emotional and mental digestive processes. It says, 'No, I no longer need this, good riddance!' It can consciously bring processes to their conclusion. It is the authority that liberates us from all behavioural patterns, convictions and belief systems which have no validity for our current situation. The large intestine meridian is a master of the art of letting go.

But if the large intestine meridian doesn't do its bidding, our convictions and beliefs will blithely continue to ferment in the darkest corners of our subconscious, and their fumes will cloud our perception, thinking and acting. We will let ourselves be influenced by excrement belonging to the past and will thus lose the freedom for conscious manoeuvring. Nonetheless, the large intestine meridian will cling to the past, since clinging is one of its core competences. However, when imbalanced, it loses the ability to discern what should be kept and what should be disposed of. It mixes up letting go with clinging, and clinging with letting go.

A healthy life principle of the large intestine meridian holds on to that which is of value. It is able to preserve and retain what is meaningful. It can build up resources. This includes dealing skilfully with material matters. To be precise, we're talking about money here, about squandering it and about laying golden eggs. If the large intestine is strong, there will always be a sufficient stash of usable leftovers. But if it is weak, there will be feelings of insecurity that there could come a day when there isn't enough. The large intestine will tense up, and this tension will, in turn, lead to obsessive clinging. Every possible effort is made to keep things under control; a ramrod rigidity sets in, the paralysing rod of fear in the backside. But this is exactly the kind of situation that requires some slack and letting go. Here, too, a firm 'no' can be helpful: 'No way!'

Saying 'no' helps to stay true to oneself and to stick to one's goals. Saying 'no' sharpens the focus. Saying 'no' reduces any distractions; it keeps the refuse outside. Saying 'no' leads to positive control and authority. Saying 'no' without feeling guilty, without being scared, without sucking up to people: that's the goal and a sign of a healthy life principle of the large intestine. This is something we're not spoon-fed. Saying 'no' must be learned, just like conscious sphincter control.

The Large Intestine Meridian and the Body

Being Fed Up

In both TCM and Western medicine, the large intestine controls the elimination of stools. However, it is not only the lower end of the gastrointestinal tract that can be blocked but also the nose. The nose has a close connection to the life principle of the large intestine and tends to be often stuffed up when it's difficult to say 'no', when a person is scared to press their point, when there is so much fear that they would rather mess their pants than open their mouth.

Other people can sense this and, unfortunately, they often see this as a welcome invitation to get precisely up the sensitive nose of someone who already finds it difficult to defend themselves, and give them a good run around or snatch something right from under their noses. It's understandable that, sooner or later, this would get up a person's nose. But instead of banging the door shut right in these people's nosy and pushy noses, you retreat timidly and tensely even further into your shell, which typically finds its expression along the pathway of the large intestine meridian.

The sinuses are the weak link in people with an imbalanced large intestine meridian. That's where it will show if something has got up your nose. The sinuses will become susceptible to chronic catarrh or inflammation since the 'no' of the large intestine meridian is connected to the immune system: immunity is our defence. It is a 'no' against pernicious influences, be they bacteria, viruses, emotional attacks or malicious opinions. A good immune system can defend itself; a weak large intestine will fail. If you can't fight well, you must at least defend yourself well.

In other words: up with the drawbridge and make sure all windows and doors are firmly shut. That would include another equally important entry to our body – the mouth. The mouth can clearly signal a defensive attitude from afar. The barely recognisable lips fiercely guard the small passage, pressed hard together with grim determination, almost devoid of blood, and as thin as the blade of a knife. Nothing and no one would be able to get through. All around, things are very tense. When speaking, there are barely any facial expressions. The voice is nasal and low. All resonance chambers are clogged up. With such people, there is a sense that one has to coax every word out of them. The face is like a rigid mask expressing distance, scepticism and cynicism, along with an arrogant know-it-all attitude. The body language signals a clear 'no'.

It's not easy to get up the noses of people like that, especially since they carry their noses too high anyway. Their potential weak points are allowing someone to come close and accepting them. Because they can't see beyond the tip of their nose. Saying 'no' too often constrains and shows up in the further course of the large intestine meridian: the chin tucked in, the shoulders pulled up, the hands closed in a fist, the buttocks tensed up. These are all precautionary measures. And as caution requires control, that's how people like that come across: reserved, uptight and with increased muscle tone. Should you still manage to get a bit closer, they will scrunch up their nose and be annoyed. A weakness in the large intestine meridian can result in chronic rhinitis, which in turn will keep others at a distance. People like that will see this as another good reason to take leave of absence from life yet again. The 'no' to life is lived by way of withdrawal and isolation because people are constantly fearful that someone may put their nose out of joint, or that they may have some other form of mishap.

In other people, however, the mouth may resemble an unmotivated opening, which flaccidly protrudes from the face. Puffy lips give in to gravity, the jaw joints appear worn. This scenario sends the message: 'All welcome! Don't worry about any security checks, you won't be searched. Help yourself, or just pass through. Just take what you need, we won't say "no" whatever you take.' The life principle of the large intestine is more like a plastic butter knife instead of a protective sword. This is a situation that can quickly lead to the nose being blocked, to be generally fed up. And there will be a tendency to play the classic role of the victim. People like that let themselves be pushed around. They are docile beings who don't put up any resistance.

Both scenarios are less than perfect for the large intestine meridian. Saying 'no' too often isolates people from life. Saying 'no' too infrequently means they can't put up any resistance. Either way, they will be fed up and their noses will be stuffed up: they don't even want to catch a whiff of life; they become tired and listless. They turn into a 'no' on two legs.

SYMPTOMS ASSOCIATED WITH THE LARGE INTESTINE MERIDIAN

Impaired nasal breathing, chronic catarrh, chronic sinusitis, nasal polyps, frequent rhinitis, increased mucous secretion, tense occiput, tense shoulders...

The Worst Is Yet to Come

The life principle of the large intestine directly manifests in the final phase of the digestive process: the worst comes at the end. We can learn a lot about the large intestine by how it deals with the ingested food that has already passed through all the other digestive organs. It tells us a lot about its strengths and weaknesses. If we can't let go, we tend to be a constipated type. If we can't hold on, we tend to be a diarrhoea type. And if we can't say 'no', we tend to be a pain type. But let's take one thing at a time...

Have you ever heard of the 'shy pooper'? These are people who can only have an easy bowel movement within the safe space of their own home because only the familiar environment allows them to let go. Mistrust and 'no' come, after all, from the same family. People like that cultivate reserve and control. This attitude can be a perfectly profitable strategy. If eating is an act of taking in, then emptying your bowels is a gesture of giving. People suffering from constipation are often prone to giving only very grudgingly. They want to hold on to what is theirs. The large intestine meridian doesn't only say 'no, that's not for me', it also says 'no, that's not for you'. And if people elevate holding on into a supreme discipline, they tend to approach life by revering stable values. This begins with an iron will for saving up and ends with greed and avarice. An exaggerated life principle of the large intestine meridian results in money spinners, who poop money until they're filthy rich. Such people just have a way with money. For them it doesn't seem to stink. They are good with material things. But they are not good with other people.

That's because strict and constraining inhibition is not good for our health in the long run, on either a physical or an emotional level. An imbalance of the large intestine energy can result in fear of letting go, and over time, not letting go will result in fully fledged stagnation. Stagnation prevents regeneration, because regeneration is always a dynamic exchange. Without regeneration, there will eventually be decay and decomposition while being alive. One can hear it, one can smell it. It begins in the guts and ends in the head. Sulphuric gases, ammonia – the devil's perfume envelops the bloated belly of the spasmodic clinger-oner. The body is poisoned, and so are the thoughts. Eventually, the head is filled with a huge heap of foetid refuse: negativity, cynicism, obsessive control, a claim to power, jealousy, resentment. Some neat and dapper diarrhoea, in the sense of a good clear-out, could here provide great relief. Because diarrhoea means letting go. Diarrhoea signals the end of restraint.

And restraint is, in turn, the end of chronic diarrhoea, which is a sign of being unable to hold on to anything. It's a loss of control; everything flows, as in early childhood when the nappies are full to overflowing. It's like being a little kid again, soiling one's pants, scared and unsure about life. The development of the life principle of the large intestine meridian has come to a standstill. If the digestive mash passes through the intestines too quickly, fluids and vital electrolytes can't be absorbed from the stool, which is too liquid. If this situation becomes chronic, it can lead to deficiency symptoms. The body loses strength, it dries out, as do the spirit and the heart, because being unable to keep anything in manifests on all levels. And if nothing can be kept in, there will eventually be emptiness.

Life will simply march right through such people. They lack the ability to stop the flow and to pick and choose what is needed. Too little of what is nourishing remains. If the life principle of the large intestine is weak, it can be difficult to build something up over a long period of time, be it prosperity, security or stability. Diarrhoea instead of golden eggs. What's lacking is the ability to stick with something, as well as self-control and the strength for holding on.

All this is lacking in people who suffer from irritable bowel syndrome. In addition, they don't have the strength to say 'no'. Without a clear 'no', there are no boundaries, and without boundaries, it's easy to become overwhelmed. Undue strain affects not only the psyche but also the intestines. After all both parties are engaged in a vivid exchange through a network of nerve fibres and neurotransmitters. If the head is overburdened, often so are the bowels, which, in turn, become irritated. It's all too much and no longer possible to digest. The nerves are raw, and the result is extreme sensitivity. There may be bloating after a meal, or there may be diarrhoea, or also constipation. This overflow has to be stopped. But how? With a feisty 'no'!

SYMPTOMS ASSOCIATED WITH THE LARGE INTESTINE MERIDIAN

Sluggish bowel movements, chronic constipation, bloating and gas, often loose stools, chronic diarrhoea, irritable bowel syndrome (IBS), ulcerative colitis...

The Large Intestine Meridian and the Psyche

Beliefs and the Past

Not every bowel movement results in a complete evacuation, and in unfavourable circumstances a lot of contaminated waste can accumulate in the colon, sometimes as much as a few kilogrammes. We may thus be carrying around a murky residue which is not only of no benefit to our metabolism but rather dangerous for our health on all levels. Faecal matter trapped in intestinal pockets corresponds to fixed convictions in the brain. Faecal matter and opinions, well preserved in our bodies, are an expression of an imbalanced large intestine meridian.

Rigidly preserved opinions often result in an equally rigid attitude towards life. Sticking to what is known is preferable to the unknown; constancy is better than change. A rather conservative attitude can over time lead to a hardening of someone's character and behaviour. Like faeces stuck for too long in the intestinal tract, devoid of any lifeblood. In other words: bone-dry, cemented into place – a solid job, a solid shirt, a solid house, a solid relationship, solid values, solid stools, solid large intestine energy. While all this provides security and guidance, in the long run it's extremely exhausting when all one's energy is used for propping up such a fake stability, come what may. But that's precisely what large intestine people want, especially and above all with regard to the future. No other meridian energy is so focussed on retirement pensions or liable to taking out all kinds of insurance policies. The large intestine loves saving accounts and taking precautions. It likes to provide for contingencies, particularly those of a material nature. If confronted with a potential threat, the large intestine is likely to soil its pants.

The large intestine meridian may therefore be obsessed with wanting, or even needing, to control everything. This is just a cover-up for the fear of not being up to the unpredictability of life by simply going with the flow. For this reason, a poorly developed large intestine doesn't like to let go; its capacity for clinging on is unparalleled, which means that the backpack of people like that is getting increasingly full. The past is carried into the present, but not everything we take from the past makes sense in the here and now. Many convictions and beliefs held a long time ago were only crutches to process certain sections of our personal development back then. Dutiful and conformist behaviour can be an important strategy during childhood to secure the parents' attention and goodwill. But if this kind of behaviour is still adhered to during adulthood, it will lead to recurring problems in a dog-eat-dog society – and it will be taken advantage of. Of course, people will always blame others because they still believe that behaviour A will lead to reaction B. Perhaps this was the case once upon a time; perhaps this was helpful a few decades ago. When the large intestine meridian is imbalanced, it's difficult to get rid of the ghosts once called upon. The belief in such rules tends to be so deeply engrained that they cannot be simply eliminated. They really are more than simple rules, but rather have the character of tenets or belief systems, which are predominantly governed by the life principle of the large intestine meridian.

Part of these belief systems is not only learned but also acquired convictions – for example, those of the parents. Anyone who was told that they were lacking any kind of talent and were unlikely to ever have any success will believe this and unerringly steer towards precisely the kind of experiences that will confirm this opinion. The scope of our belief systems determines the range of our perceptions and experiences. Even if they are not really conducive to our well-being, they are like stuck digestive residue, a part of our personality which we cannot easily dispense with.

An imbalance of the life principle of the large intestine can lead to exaggerated clinging to obsolete patterns, values or opinions, even to fanatical and missionary behaviours, like an intestinal obstruction on a psychological level. Everything stagnates. And this stagnation can lead to proliferation or inflammation. Big religious wars can be triggered by the most trivial issues. Often a tiny spark is enough to kindle a blaze. What could be of help here? Applying the principle of cleansing the bowels on all levels: purging, flushing, letting go, evacuating. An enema for body, mind and spirit. A thorough cleanse to eliminate all concretions and incrustations from the body. A 'no' to all the echoes from the past that are no longer needed. A 'yes' to the self and to the person you truly are.

Guilt, Obsession and Perfectionism

What is the large intestine meridian particularly sensitive to? Feelings of guilt! Because it likes to carry with it stuff from the past, particularly belief systems and moral values, preferably those of important caregivers, first and foremost the parents. They stick! They're like a subtle moral authority observing independent actions from the depths of the guts and putting them into context with what has been internalised a long time ago, mainly during early childhood development. This can easily lead to moral conflicts. People can feel caught out acting against deep-seated convictions. The inner 'that's not the done thing' voice is chipping away at their self-confidence, a bad conscience begins to surface, and the resulting feelings of guilt are strong enough to force the strongest 'no' to its knees. There is the desire to conform and not to disappoint. If the large intestine meridian is weak, people feel guilty easily and quickly. One wry look can be enough to lead you to cross-examine yourself for hours about what you may have done wrong this time round. Being late for work once can be enough to make you feel bad for weeks.

The tension caused by not wanting to disappoint can lead to

another idiosyncrasy of the large intestine meridian: perfectionism. Perfectionism is the polar opposite of the free and chaotic run of events. Perfectionism means to have everything under control, especially oneself. Letting go and relaxing is completely out of the question. No, I'm not good enough. No, this was too little. No, this could be better. All this is a cover-up for the fear that things may not go well – for example, one's life plans. If this fear is big, the large intestine meridian will rise to the occasion. It will conscientiously, dutifully and ambitiously stick to actions and rules that serve the sole purpose of fulfilling the highest moral values and approaching an almost immaculate self-image. People like that don't want to feel disgusted by what's coming out the other end. The natural rhythm of holding on and letting go is disturbed: control has gained control of control.

This represents yet again a condition of utter blockage towards life. Nothing flows any more without a person's volition. Healthy large intestine energy is perfectly able to flow but doesn't have to. It can pull itself together if circumstances require this. It can force itself, it can control itself, and, indeed, now and again this is crucially necessary. It can rein in fear and curb insecurity. It can subdue chaos and create order. Its ability to hold on is superb, even when the storms of life are rattling the foundations. Without these abilities of the large intestine, bigger challenges, outstanding achievements and existential crises could hardly be managed. A well-integrated life principle of the large intestine meridian even has a predilection for perfection. It loves completion. It can stubbornly pursue some issue, not for the sake of conforming or seeking attention, but as an expression of a natural process that has been optimised for as long as necessary to reach its maximum potential. Just as the large intestine represents the completion of digestion.

Signs of an Imbalanced and Balanced Large Intestine Meridian

Signs of an Imbalanced Large Intestine Meridian

- Tendency to bloating, fullness, diarrhoea, constipation, irritable bowel syndrome

- Delicate nasal passages and sinuses

  Poor stamina, things easily slipping from one's grasp
- Can be easily manipulated, weak boundaries, often feelings of guilt
- Not good at dealing with material matters
- Tendency to compulsive control and perfectionism
- High muscle tone, poor flexibility, stiffness

Signs of a Balanced Large Intestine Meridian

- Good digestion, robust immunity
- Healthy boundaries, good at managing conflicts
- Dealing well with material matters and money
- Ability to let go and find closure
- Striving for perfection and high standards
- Stamina based on perseverance and tenacity

How to Strengthen the Life Principle of the Large Intestine Meridian

Saying 'No'

Take one day each week when you respond with a friendly but unambiguous 'no' to the idea of having to get it right for everybody. Avoid phrases such as 'rather not', 'a bit inconvenient' or 'yes, but'. Go for a loud and clear 'no'. Look the person right in the eye. Support the 'no' with a slight shake of the head and appropriate hand gestures. Be clear: you really mean this. For this reason, also omit any form of justification. Any form of explanation provides an opening for attempts at persuasion. Don't offer such potential targets! Should you find it really difficult to say 'no' to big challenges, request some time for consideration and communicate your 'no' digitally. No. Thank you. And without a burst of justification. Say 'no' to unpleasant tasks, 'no' to pointless activities, 'no' to uninspiring chats, 'no' to well-meant but interfering attempts to distract you, and 'no' to chatterboxes and energy vampires. Say 'no' without feeling guilty. Discover the joy of saying 'no'. Because each 'no' harbours a 'yes' to yourself.

Recognising Belief Systems

Give yourself one week to recognise and get a sense of your belief systems and convictions. Pay attention to generalisations in your thought patterns and your use of language – for example, 'everybody', 'always', 'it's the done thing', 'it can't be done like that'. Are there any particular phrases that are often used in your family ('only the strong survive', 'no pain, no gain', 'everything is getting more expensive')? Do you recognise the patterning of your parents or other people close to you in the way you think and act? Try to understand why your parents or caregivers developed these patterns. Look at old family photographs, old pictures from school. What kind of values were suggested to you and by whom? What kind of convictions were you exposed to in your past? What has this got to do with you? Try to extract the three most frequent beliefs and convictions having an effect on your life. Write them down. Write down in which aspect of your life they have the biggest impact. And then reflect: Are these patterns useful or inhibiting? If they inhibit you: How could you rephrase these convictions so that they are more appropriate to your current life plans?

The Pathway of the Large Intestine Meridian

The large intestine meridian begins with Large Intestine 1 at the thumb-side of the index finger. From Large Intestine 1, it follows the thumb-side of the index finger on the line 'between the palmar and dorsal aspects' to the base joint of the index finger. It continues along the second metacarpal bone to Large Intestine 4, a prominent point on the bulge that forms by pressing the thumb against the hand. When abducting the thumb, a depression forms at the wrist crease. This is the location of Large Intestine 5, the so-called anatomical snuff box.

From Large Intestine 5, the large intestine meridian follows the radius along the forearm. It crosses the long abductor pollicis longus muscle, and then courses along the thumb-side of two important hand extensors, the extensor carpi radialis longus and brevis, all the way to Large Intestine 11, which can be found in a depression that forms at the thumb-side end of the elbow crease when the elbow is flexed.

From Large Intestine 11, the meridian ascends the upper arm to Large Intestine 14, located halfway up the upper arm at the tip of the insertion of the deltoid. The large intestine meridian then runs between the middle and anterior heads of the deltoid to Large Intestine 15, which can be found below the protrusion of the collarbone (clavicle). Continuing from Large Intestine 15, the meridian courses to a depression formed by the spine of the scapula and the collarbone.

It then follows the anterior border of the trapezius, running at a distance of a thumb-width roughly parallel to the curved contour of the clavicle. Superior to the lateral insertion of the sternocleidomastoid muscle, it ascends to Large Intestine 18, traversing the anterior lateral aspect of the neck. This point is located three thumb-widths lateral to the laryngeal cartilage. After crossing the lower jaw, approximately one thumb-width from the mandibular angle, it then diagonally traverses the lower cheek directly towards Large Intestine 20 at the upper border of the depression lateral to the nasal wing.

Key Areas of the Large Intestine Meridian

Nose, Neck and Shoulders

The large intestine meridian terminates directly below the nose at the point Large Intestine 20, *ying xiang* or 'Welcome Fragrance'. This point indicates whether 'our nose is full up', as the German phrase has it, meaning that we are fed up, or whether we are easily annoyed. Or perhaps we think life stinks and respond with a 'no' in the form of a blocked nose. A blocked nose impairs inhalation, and thus also affects the life principle of the lungs, because our sense of smell also represents our instinct. A keen sense of smell can help to pick up and pursue even subtle scents. But if we lack this trait, we rely less on our feelings and more on the power of our reason. Control instead of intuition.

This can also be apparent on the section of the large intestine meridian on the neck. The neck becomes stiff. It is retracted. We lose the connection to heaven, to the expansiveness of life, to new horizons. We're stuck, both in our convictions and in our 'this is how it has to be' mentality. This attitude is expressed in the point Large Intestine 17, 'Heaven's Tripod' or *tian ding*. *Ding* also refers to an offering cup, represented here by the skull resting on the spinal column and the two muscular cords formed by the sternocleido-mastoid. When the cup is full, it can't receive anything new. It needs to be emptied. If our skull is filled with rigid beliefs and values, we become hard-headed, unable to look left or right. This may well be mirrored in a high muscle tone of the neck as well as a limited range of motion. The skull needs to be emptied.

This chain of tension, of refusal and of saying 'no' often continues all the way to Large Intestine 15, *jian yu* or 'Shoulder Bone'. The question in this area is whether we are carrying a weight on our shoulders or whether we are able to take things easy. From a TCM perspective, many shoulder problems originate in the large intestine meridian. Hunched shoulders can be a sign of self-protection when we are unable to verbalise and squeeze out a 'no', instead internalising it so that it becomes stuck in the body. The burden of the past, the burden of too much responsibility, the burden of life all push down on us and limit our scope for action.

Elbows

The area around the elbows is the origin of the major part of the forearm musculature. The elbows are the seat of the strength for holding on and letting go. And it's the location for one of the most important points on the large intestine meridian: Large Intestine 11, *qu chi* or the 'Pool at the Crook'. In TCM, this point is used as a so-called ghost point, a point with a direct connection to the psyche. Large Intestine 11 is located right within the forearm extensors. By extending the muscles on the forearm, we let go. In acupuncture,

Large Intestine 11 is a popular point for treating constipation. It is also indicated for diarrhoea since we are unable to hold anything. We can't hold on to things; it's all just slipping through our fingers. The area around Large Intestine 11 generally tends to be quite sensitive. It's the origin of many cases of tendinitis, generally a symptom of overstraining. The 'no' wasn't said in time, either to oneself or to others. With our elbows sticking out, we define the boundary of our space; we get our way. This, too, mirrors the life principle of the large intestine meridian.

Index Fingers

A raised index finger represents a loud and clear 'no!' It can be considered a drawn sword, used to defend but also to control. Furthermore, of all the fingers, the index finger is the strongest when it comes to holding on: it is predestined to cling on. Not without reason, the large intestine meridian begins on the index finger. The strongest point in this region is Large Intestine 4, *he gu* or 'Joining Valley', between the thumb and index finger. As the source point of the large intestine meridian, it is a point which influences the energy of the entire meridian. Large Intestine 4 is one of the strongest points for letting go in TCM.

By clenching a fist, Large Intestine 4 rises conspicuously between thumb and index finger, like a little mountain. Holding on in an exaggerated manner, things start to accumulate, just like a mountain. Large Intestine 4 ensures that these accumulations pour down into the valley, regardless of whether they manifest in the shoulders ('carrying the weight of the world on one's shoulders'), in the face ('clenching one's teeth') or in someone's digestion ('having a rod up one's backside'). To avoid such a situation in the first place, it can be of benefit to draw your sword now and again and sever all the constricting knots.

The Large Intestine Meridian: Key Points

- Associated element: Metal element
- Quality: Yang
- Time on the organ clock: 5am–7am
- Animal quality: Rabbit
- Partner meridian: Lung meridian
- Twinned meridian: Stomach meridian
- Opposite meridian: Kidney meridian

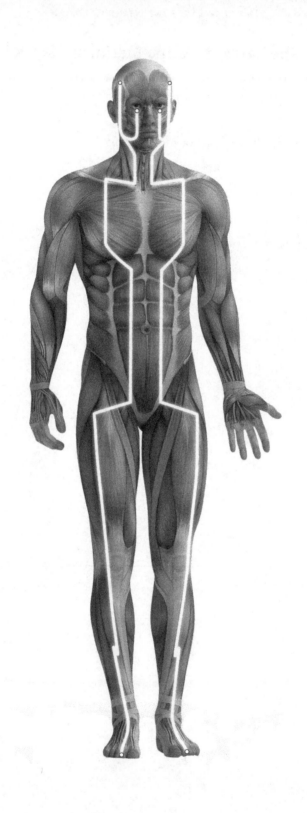

Chapter 5

The Stomach Meridian
The Art of Hunting

Questions for the Stomach Meridian

- Do I have a good appetite for life? Am I curious about life?
- Do I take from the smorgasbord of life what makes me full and content?
- Am I able to nourish myself independently and consciously? Financially? Emotionally? Mentally?
- Do I have the necessary edge to get my way?
- Am I able to pursue a goal with focus and tenacity?
- Is it easy for me to digest input, both information and emotions?
- Am I easily peeved?
- Do I have the courage to leave my comfort zone, again and again, in order to experience new things?
- Am I able to process things and bring them 'down to earth'?

The Life Principle of the Stomach Meridian

When we are hungry, the stomach meridian gets active. Its task is to make us full. It fills the hole in our tummy. It fills the hole in our hearts. It fills the hole in our soul. It goes hunting and gets what we are lacking. The stomach meridian is our hunter, and good hunters need a wide range of skills. They need focus, determination and stamina. They need to know what they are after. They need to be able to gauge whether they can cope with the prey they want to kill. They have to pounce at the right time, they have to be able to bring the prey home and they have to be able to process it. When a hunter is able to do all these things, there will always be a richly laden table. There will be no scarcity, no hunger, no unfulfilled needs. Abundance instead of emptiness. It is the life principle of the stomach meridian to make sure our system is sufficiently provided for – on all levels.

Integrating the life principle of the stomach meridian represents an important step in our development. It represents the exodus from paradise, the renunciation of the protective mother's breast. When the teeth break through, the stomach meridian experiences a developmental boost. It's a leap towards autonomy, towards activity. At the same time, there is an increase in the ability to process the larger lumps served by life, whether these are food or new challenges. Life means confrontation, and confrontation needs the strength to bite back. Welcome to the wild; welcome to the real world. And the real world may give you a tough time. Or it may sit heavily in your stomach, like a stone.

A weak stomach meridian lacks the ability to bite back. It can deal with everyday life only in the form of mush, preferably pre-digested by others. There's no desire to chew, to shred, to process. No desire to form an opinion, to make an effort, to bother, to deal with problems. Any confrontation is a reason for bolting. What is desired is instant gratification. We never want to leave our cosy comfort zone, and live in hope that life, like a constantly available breast filled to the brim with milk and honey, will be there, hey presto, to nourish and indulge us at the slightest indisposition. It's a form of clinging on to paradise, dwelling in a time when there was nothing we had to worry about because someone else was kind enough to take care of everything.

This is a far cry from being an independent hunter; rather, it is holding on to a state of dependence. The hunting instinct is missing, as is any drive. You prefer to curb your appetite rather than set your sight on scrumptious titbits. You would rather be content with what's banged on the table right in front of you, no matter whether it's tasty or not, whether it's filling or not, whether it makes you content or not. Whether it's your plate, your job, your relationship or your life perspective, everything has to be easy to swallow and easy to process. The nutritional value for body and soul is a minor point.

This approach, however, misses the core questions of the stomach meridian: Am I able to nourish myself? Am I able to provide for myself? Am I able to pursue and achieve precisely what I need and desire for my life to be content and fulfilled? On a physical, mental, emotional and spiritual level? People with a strong stomach meridian tend to be right at the front of the queue for the smorgasbord of existence. They don't wait to be served. They are not sitting around with an empty stomach, hoping that something will happen. They go hunting, if required, with a vigour bordering on aggression. They have the necessary bite to do so. They are able to bare their teeth, able to get their teeth into something, able to bite their way through adversity. They have developed an acute sense of where something worthwhile can be found, and the ability to move there fast. They have the capacity to quickly suss out a situation and grasp it as well. They are very focussed. It's for a reason that the stomach meridian begins at the eyes, governs the mouth and the jaw, and terminates on the legs. Seeing, biting, pursuing, hunting. If you're good at all these, there will be abundance instead of scarcity. There will be a positive balance.

The Stomach Meridian and the Body

Bite and Swallow

The pathway of the stomach meridian begins at the eyes. After all, we need to assess every object of our desire before setting off to make it ours. However, the first important key section of the stomach meridian is the jaw. After all, it's no use eyeing something of value if we lack the will and self-assertion to get hold of it. The emptiness in the stomach will remain when we have to watch others happily snatch away the booty right before our eyes because we don't have the edge to snap at it ourselves at the right moment. The masticatory musculature manifests around the jaw, and this is where it becomes obvious if we are able to clench our teeth with determination and approach a target without compromise. If we're

unable to consistently follow a goal, it will be difficult to be successful. Good hunters show it in their face: a pronounced, broad chin;
jaws ditto. A biter through and through. Hungry for success and able
to get it. An excellent provider, 100% performance-driven. This is a
stomach meridian with a well-developed life principle.

Those able to care well for themselves could, in theory, also care
well for others. That's why this type of physiognomy is generally
considered attractive, especially in men. The problem: good hunters
are primarily concerned with themselves and often can't get enough.
What took a lot of toil to get, they want to keep, while those who
share may go empty-handed at the end of the day. Therefore: 'no' to
giving, 'yes' to taking. All mine. Relinquishing is not a feature of the
stomach meridian, and even less so of an overactive stomach meridian. It likes to push itself prominently into the foreground, the same
way people with aggressive stomach energy like to push their chin
forward. This sends a clear signal: pugnacity and dominance. Often,
conspicuous jaws transition into equally prominent hamster-like
cheeks: a storage area, emergency rations for bad times. Provide
and be prepared. Your need for prosperity needs to be safeguarded.
Your own, and not that of others! A tense stomach meridian tends
to manifest in a pronounced selfishness. The daily mantra is 'me,
me, me'. We're always ready to bare our teeth to defend our prey
and territory. If others are in the way of our needs, we are ready to
devour them. In our aspirations for life and for ourselves, we can
be like a terrier with its teeth stuck in a bone. We are big-mouthed,
and we bite off more than we can chew because we are scared of
not getting enough, not enough nourishment for our souls – that
is, attention and recognition.

If the life principle of the stomach meridian is weak, the jaws
hang down slackly. Even when life passes right under our nose, we
don't get the idea that we should make a move and treat ourselves
to a tasty bite. There just isn't enough edge to our teeth. It seems
preferable to run away from any challenge rather than facing it. This
attitude seems to prevail in people with a receding chin that seems
to withdraw from the face. It's as if their chin is trying to hide in
order not to provoke a confrontation. Their masseter (masticatory
muscle) is weak, their jaw feeble: no assertiveness whatsoever. Providing provisions is a great worry. Instead of pouch-like hamster

cheeks, the face is gaunt: a deficiency that is difficult to reverse since poor stomach energy results in little hunger for life. And when there is no hunger, why go hunting? After all, we're content with the morsels left behind by others at the buffet. We prefer the cheap seats, or we may not even show up. A lack of appetite for our own existence. The ego structure is only poorly developed, coupled with weak assertiveness. Subservience rather than dominance. A scavenger rather than a hunter.

Furthermore, our ability to take a hearty bite and chew with gusto reflects how we deal with the tough cookies life may throw at us. If we feel that we can't cope with them, it seems sensible to avoid them straight away; otherwise, they may sit in our stomach like a stone, sometimes for years. Flight instead of hunting, especially when emotions are involved, especially when it's about resentment and discontent. And if evading a confrontation doesn't work, emotional stuff gets swallowed without resistance, but also without further processing. Because the tasks of the stomach meridian include breaking down everything that enters our system from the outside, not just food and fluids but also, and in particular, emotions, information and encounters. All these require recording, processing and dissecting into little pieces in order to turn them into something else. That is true digestion.

A strong stomach meridian can break down even the heartiest of bites. Nothing – not even stuff that's really hard to digest, like a recalcitrant dumpling – will get stuck in the throat, an area traversed by the stomach meridian. Whatever is taken in will slip down smoothly, sufficiently macerated, ready to be further metabolised and eliminated. Such people are not scared of conflicts or resistance, they don't shy away from arguments, because they know that they are able to process even unpleasant things.

However, without the required processing, the stomach can become easily upset – an upset stomach, so to speak – since it doesn't have the appropriate response to deal with the stuff accumulating inside it. It desperately nibbles away without anything actually happening. It becomes fuller and fuller. It's constantly peeved. The corners of the mouth, also situated on the pathway of the stomach meridian, droop listlessly downwards. No wonder we begin to lose our appetite. No wonder the stomach is quick to respond with an acid attitude, and that, by belching to the point of vomiting, it tries to bring to the surface all the undigested things as a reminder of the loose ends lying dormant deep within our bodies. No wonder there is gnashing of teeth, especially during the night, when the sleep-induced relaxation opens the gate to our subconscious and our bodies try to process and digest what has been left behind during the day.

If the life principle of the stomach meridian is well developed, it provides us with a healthy zest and good appetite for life, along with the ability to process and assimilate what has been taken in so as to make good use of it. A well-developed life principle endows us with the strength and confidence of a successful hunter who knows they're capable of providing for themselves.

SYMPTOMS ASSOCIATED WITH THE STOMACH MERIDIAN

Tension in the jaw, bruxism, lockjaw, inflammation of the gums, difficulty swallowing, the feeling of a lump in one's throat, belching, fullness sensations, loss of appetite, hyperacidity...

Constant Grounding

A good hunter needs one thing in particular: good legs. It doesn't suffice to be hungry in order to get full. There will come a point when you have to start moving in order to satisfy your needs. The pathway of the stomach meridian connects the legs and feet with the eyes and the jaw. Seeing, registering, getting hooked by the target, sprinting: it's for a reason that the stomach meridian controls the strongest thigh muscle, the quadriceps, so well defined in most runners. When the legs are strong, even the most persistent prey is fit for pursuit. Stay with it, further and even further, as fast as possible. That's what a strong stomach meridian can do. Hunger is its fuel, greed its engine. Obstacles will be overrun, barriers broken. You need stamina and steadiness until you can eventually pounce. It requires continuous striding forth.

A tired stomach meridian, however, lacks the drive even to raise itself out of the chair called cosiness. Its hunting ground is its comfort zone, and this tends to be rather restricted. Everything outside of its habitual environment appears dangerous and is therefore not aspired to. Appetite for new experiences is limited or completely lacking. Making do with little as a stopgap. Retirement as life purpose. Stamina: absent. Not standing up to one's needs. Not facing difficulties. No progress. Fear of the big wide world. Being stuck in the crawling phase of life and the small radius of action that comes with it. Weak legs that are a far cry from serving as the mainstay of one's identity. Poor grounding.

Poor grounding also occurs when the connecting function of the stomach meridian is imbalanced, especially when the digestion of non-material things, primarily information, is affected. Information has to be processed, just like food, and therefore it falls within the remit of the stomach meridian. Information has to be taken in and reduced to small pieces so that it can be processed and be of use to us. People with a strong stomach meridian are quick as well as effective thinkers. In TCM, the stomach is seen as the seat of reason. It ensures a high capacity for mental processing. It instantly recognises whether a piece of information is essential or not; it is good at analysing and categorising; at dissecting everything and picking it apart down to the most minute detail. And the stomach meridian is actually able to do something worthwhile with the knowledge thus gained: it can implement it directly and without any delay. It can bring thoughts down to earth. The connection between the head and the legs functions well. This corresponds to the natural direction of flow of the stomach meridian: from above to below.

If thoughts knocked out of the sky can't reach the ground, they get stuck in the skull. I think, therefore I am – excessive mental masturbation can be an expression of the stomach energy being out of balance. There is much intense thinking without any tangible results. Much is made out of little. What's lacking is good grounding. Also lacking is the kind of processing that yields results. These are cerebral people who live their lives in their heads. They're obstinate when it comes to thinking. Their entire energy is concentrated in the brain. It can become dangerous when there is too much mental digesting to be done; it leads to infobesity. Such information overload isn't any different from an overly hearty mental meal exceeding our capacity for processing. When we overeat, the food will fester in our stomach. It's for a reason that a person who is exposed to a continuous flow of dense information, whether generated externally or internally, tends to have a very sensitive stomach. It can easily run hot if it can't keep up with its task of processing, which can then lead to it being overloaded. Nothing else can fit in. Initially, there will be only sour belching, but sooner or later the stomach may become inflamed: Hello, heartburn! Hello, gastritis! Yet for many people this is still no reason to tread more carefully, and the condition can become chronic. Furthermore, people will start to lose the ground beneath their feet: their grounding. There will be a separation of body and mind. There will be thinking instead of feeling. There is no longer body awareness. And people become even more stubborn. What would help in such cases is a light, easy-to-digest diet, alighting from the mental merry-go-round, gradually reducing all the things that have to be processed. Making less out of too much. Less thinking, more doing.

In the context of the stomach meridian, grounding means to complete something, bring it down to earth, create results, ensure the availability of tangible provisions. Implementing a small idea has often more nutritional value than ten thousand daydreams whirring through the sky. Indeed, this tends to be the problem of an overactive or overwhelmed stomach meridian: continuously hunting for new things. By doing so, it's easy to get lost. Therefore, the task of the leg section of the stomach meridian is to provide good purchase to the ground to avoid getting lost in one's mental world.

SYMPTOMS ASSOCIATED WITH THE STOMACH MERIDIAN

Weakness in the legs, lack of stamina, fatigue, lack of motivation, heartburn, gastritis, emotional overwhelm, excessive thinking...

The Stomach Meridian and the Psyche

Hunger and Appetite

It's never a good idea to go shopping when you're hungry. Hunger is an existential need, a signal for survival. Hunger is the result of an energy deficit and is defined as a motivational state for the procurement of food as well as its ingestion. This is precisely what the stomach meridian stands for: if there is a deficit, it needs to be balanced. The hole in the stomach needs to be plugged, by hook or by crook. With true hunger, selection mechanisms are put on the back burner, while impulsive as well as instinctive behaviours take the helm. Hunger means feeding, means now, means anything at all. Hunger means needs must. It's a completely different matter with appetite. Appetite is about wanting. Appetite is conscious selection. Appetite is liking something. Appetite is learned and influenced by early-childhood impressions, habits, psychological sensitivities or cultural idiosyncrasies. Hunger versus appetite. Glutton versus gourmet. Hunger is stronger than appetite. That's the problem the stomach meridian has to deal with.

The stomach meridian is responsible for balancing the supplies on all levels: physically, mentally, emotionally, spiritually. On balance, there should be a slight surplus. Or, rather, a contentment that gives hunger a tough time, allows appetite to roam freely and ensures that we make conscious choices about what we ingest. On a physical level, it's not all that hard for the stomach meridian: our living conditions are such that we don't experience hunger. We have the luxury and the freedom to make choices based on our appetite, even if many decisions related to our diet aren't always the best.

But what about our hunger on a mental and emotional level? Here, too, we have to hunt for what makes us content. But what if we have never really learned how to do this? If we have never adequately integrated the life principle of the stomach meridian? If we are not able to nourish ourselves with love, attention and meaning, maturely and self-responsibly? Then the hunger remains. And hunger takes it all. Without batting an eyelid, it takes the first available partner promising to fill the emptiness of its heart, even if only a little bit. As long as this promise stands, we will love that person to bits. However, when disillusion sets in, we are eaten up by frustration and are fed up with our hastily chosen partner – often for years, often for the rest of our lives. Or we choose a profession for which we are willing to sell our soul if that gets us a bit of attention. We're willing to give everything for a little bit of recognition because our hunger for it is huge. We don't choose according to our appetite and what we would really like, but with a sense of 'needs must'.

Sometimes the stomach meridian may try to compensate for the hunger felt on one level with abundance on another: chocolate instead of lovesickness. A luxury holiday instead of searching for meaning. Status symbols instead of self-worth. The problem: any deficit has to be resolved on the correct level. Balancing an emotional or mental hole with material abundance won't work in the long run. The hole will remain. And the stomach meridian will keep running and running and running. Until it runs out of steam. Excess on the one hand and a gaping void on the other. We are choking on our possessions while our happiness is on the breadline. But happiness insists on being nourished. In the desperate attempt to fill the hole in the soul, we devour pretty much everything the fridge or the biscuit tin has to offer. Again and again and again. Many eating disorders, from food cravings to bulimia, have their roots in an imbalanced stomach meridian. Or the inner emptiness may be expressed by refusing food. Look at me, my heart is starving, doesn't anyone notice? I want to be fed with love, filled with recognition!

If the stomach gets bogged down by its task of finding the right balance of how much to ingest, it's necessary to say 'Stop!' This situation requires a person to do an open, honest and thorough inventory of the larder that is their life: What is really missing? What do I need to be full and content on the appropriate level? When this has been achieved, the stomach meridian has to be put on the right scent. The solution is self-sufficiency. To love oneself. To pay attention to oneself. To give meaning to oneself. Only once most of the hunger has been stilled will appetite arise. The stomach meridian stands for the hunger for life. Hunger is its obligation, appetite its embellishment. And when both come together and complement each other, only then will the life principle of the stomach have truly matured.

Curiosity, Greed and Egoism

A well-developed stomach meridian expresses itself in a keen curiosity towards life. Curiosity is like the hunter who is tempted to find out whether there may be more worthwhile prey behind that hill he has never traversed before. Departing into the unknown. Being interested in uncharted territory. Searching for new discoveries. Having appetite for further development. Curiosity is one of the most important human traits. It is the driving force for all innovation, the path to knowledge and insight. Not feeling fulfilled and content with what has been achieved already. A healthy stomach energy ensures that the invigorating quality of curiosity is maintained into old age. This will keep you young. It will keep you fresh and alert, curious like a small child with a huge appetite for life.

However, the stomach meridian, with its latent tendency towards exaggeration, can sometimes be a bit too generous with its curiosity. People who constantly go beyond their boundaries, who prefer to flirt with the unknown, may get their fingers burned now and again. And it's only a small step from curiosity to greed. Greed is the expression of an imbalanced stomach meridian which panics about never getting enough and tries to devour everything. That's evolution for you. The more game was hunted, the bigger the chance was for survival. Greed makes the stomach meridian susceptible to addictive behaviour, be it shopping, adventures or gambling. People want more, and even more isn't enough: flying round the globe 30 times, 300 pairs of shoes, £300,000 in the bank account. Constantly on the hunt.

Greed has also an egocentric overtone. Greed likes taking, and it doesn't shy away from taking from others should that be advantageous. Greed devours. Greed is beyond any moral consensus, beyond rules and regulations. Greed wants to be higher and faster, to go further. At all cost. Egomania. Regardless of the consequences. One's ego and one's needs are always central. To be the best and greatest hunter in the world. And the stomach meridian runs hot. On a physical level, there may be hyperacidity due to the never-ending running around. Heat and acidity attack the stomach lining. The flesh lies bare. Greed to the point of self-destruction. Nonetheless, it's never content and satisfied.

It seems as if a poorly developed stomach meridian has a much easier life, being indifferently stuck to the couch in the shape of a potato. No excitement, no butterflies in the stomach, no urge to explore, no curiosity, no greed. But no sign of any progress either, and even less zest. Walking through life is a rather dull affair.

Your home is your comfort zone, which you never leave unless for a very good reason. Being satisfied very quickly, without really being satisfied. But this state of affairs is not in keeping with the life principle of the stomach meridian either. The stomach meridian takes its orders from the soul. It is supposed to deliver what is fulfilling.

Signs of an Imbalanced and Balanced Stomach Meridian

Signs of an Imbalanced Stomach Meridian

- Little drive, little hunger, little appetite
- Little self-sufficiency, little autonomy, little self-responsibility, preferring to stay in one's comfort zone
- Poor stamina, weak legs
- Hyperactivity, nervousness, inner restlessness, being driven
- Egocentric world view, egoism
- Tendency to constipation, fullness sensations, gastritis, heartburn, diarrhoea
- Tendency to inflammatory gum problems, teeth grinding, tension in the jaw

Signs of a Balanced Stomach Meridian

- Good bite, good digestion, strong legs
- Good stamina and concentration, strong focus
- Capacity for emotional, mental and financial self-sufficiency
- Quick perception, good intellectual capacity
- Curiosity about and interest in progress and uncharted territory
- Comfortable with growth
- Good at implementing and doing

How to Strengthen the Life Principle of the Stomach Meridian

Am I Able to Nourish Myself?

The stomach meridian likes to chase after goals that promise contentment. But are these really your goals? What does really satisfy you? Take a week to reflect on the following questions: What makes me happy and content on a material level? What makes me happy and content emotionally? What makes me happy and content mentally?

Can you provide for these goals yourself, without developing some form of dependence or requiring help? A strong stomach meridian is able to achieve this. What about you?

Fasting

Fasting refers to any form of reduction in order to unburden our system. While fasting has many different forms, they all have one thing in common: the hyperactive hunter called stomach meridian will quickly show its true face. If it feels it's not getting enough, it panics and gets nervous. That's a sign that fasting is indicated in order to show the hunter that this won't be the end of the world; that even with less, it's possible to get full. Give yourself a week. Fast in the area where your hunter is most active. Go offline for a week. No computer, no phone. Be by yourself for a week. Don't buy anything you don't need for a week. Abstain from sweets for a week. Or stay away from all food for a week. Your stomach meridian will be grateful. Repeat week-long fasts several times a year.

The Pathway of the Stomach Meridian

The stomach meridian begins at Stomach 1, located below the pupil in the eye socket, in a slight depression of the bone. It then courses downward to Stomach 4, a bit lateral to the corner of the mouth. From Stomach 4, the stomach meridian curves laterally along the lower jaw towards Stomach 6, a point which becomes prominent by clenching the jaw: Stomach 6 is the highest point of the big masticatory muscle, the masseter. Just before reaching this point, the stomach meridian forks. One branch descends towards the neck. The other branch ascends in front of the ear from Stomach 6 to Stomach 8, located at the corner of the forehead, where the chewing action can still be felt in the temporal muscle. The second branch runs from the forking point vertically down the neck to Stomach 9. This point can be found one and a half thumb-widths from the Adam's apple on the anterior border of the sternocleidomastoid. From Stomach 9, the meridian courses to Stomach 11, located vertically below Stomach 9 on the upper border of the collar bone. The meridian continues along the upper border of the clavicle towards the shoulder to reach the point Stomach 12, roughly at the midpoint of the collar bone, vertically above the nipple. From Stomach 12, the stomach meridian descends via the nipple (Stomach 17) to the fifth intercostal space, where it veers more medially. It crosses the lower border of the ribcage at the sixth intercostal space to reach the abdomen near the point Stomach 19.

From Stomach 19, the stomach meridian courses two thumb-widths from the midline in a straight line towards the pubic bone to the point Stomach 30, located on the upper border of the pubic bone, where the inguinal pulse is clearly palpable. The meridian then traverses the hip bone in a lateral direction to Stomach 31, which can be found below the anterior superior iliac spine, at the level of the pubic symphysis. The stomach meridian continues along the thigh, in an anatomical depression between two heads (rectus femoris, vastus lateralis) of the four-headed quadriceps, towards the outer border of the kneecap (patella). It then follows the outer edge of the patella to what is probably the best-known acupuncture point of all: Stomach 36.

Stomach 36 is located three thumb-widths below the lower border of the patella and one thumb-width lateral to the tibial crest. From here, the stomach meridian courses along the tibia on the muscle belly of the tibialis anterior. Above the lateral malleolus, it begins to change direction towards the front of the ankle joint. Stomach 41 is an important landmark here, located in the middle of the horizontal crease between two clearly palpable tendons. The stomach meridian continues past the highest point of the back of the foot, the location of Stomach 42. It then courses in a depression between the second and third toes and terminates on the outer aspect of the second toe at the point Stomach 45, next to the corner of the nail.

Key Areas of the Stomach Meridian

Jaw and Neck

The mighty masseter is the muscle with the greatest leverage and, relative to its size, is the strongest muscle in our body. It is the muscle we use to bite, the muscle we use to get our teeth into something. Directly on the muscle is the point Stomach 6, *jia che* or 'Jaw Chariot'. In TCM, Stomach 6 is a so-called ghost point – that is, a point with a strong effect on and a direct connection to the psyche – since its prominence is an expression of the strength of our bite and our drive. Exaggerated doggedness is a trait that can often lead to problems. People see only themselves and nothing but themselves because the stomach has the tendency to become embroiled in the importance of its ego, to the point of jaw spasms, lockjaw or intense nocturnal teeth grinding. Relaxing the jaw musculature can resolve many mental knots: stepping back from one's own importance and personal dramas. This loosens us up, makes us more easy-going, especially in how we deal with others.

This openness reveals itself at the point Stomach 9, *ren ying* or 'Man's Welcome'. Stomach 9 governs the area of the larynx, including the thyroid. If you've got too much on your plate, it's difficult to welcome anything. If you are up to your neck, it's difficult to be open, because you're much too busy with keeping things at bay. It's difficult to say 'welcome' to new things or people around you if you constantly have a lump in your throat, or, worse, if even bigger pieces are permanently lodged there. It creates pressure, and pressure creates heat. An overactive thyroid can be related to the stomach meridian. The hunter is running hot. You're burning yourself up, and nothing much remains.

This is particularly obvious at the next key point: Stomach 12, *que pen*, 'Beggar's Hole' or 'Empty Basin'. Whether we are able to provide well for ourselves is also reflected in our physical robustness.

By observing the area around someone's collarbone, we can quickly establish whether they are suffering from deprivation or living in abundance. It's an area where trenches of hunger may open up, with sunken flesh and protruding bones.

Abdomen

Things we can't digest upset our stomach. This is expressed at Ren Mai 12, *zhong wan* or 'Middle Epigastrium'. Located on the midline of the abdomen, four thumb-widths above the navel, this is the alarm point of the stomach. In Shiatsu, it is also the diagnostic area of the pericardium meridian, the 'heart protector', whose task is to protect the heart from intense emotional strain. And what is most difficult to digest? Emotions. Emotions can sit heavily in one's stomach for years. The result: feeling too full all too quickly; a hard stomach; tension pain around Ren Mai 12. All this causes a lot of strain. The abdomen, our centre, is unable to support us. The 'Heavenly Pillar', Stomach 25 or *tian shu*, two thumb-widths lateral to the navel, groans and sighs under the burden. We have lost our middle because it is clogged up with undigested residual waste. The abdomen is therefore another area where tension and increased sensitivity may occur.

Pelvis

Our ability for grounding ourselves manifests in the flexibility of our hips. This flexibility is determined by the points Stomach 30, *qi chong* or 'Rushing Qi', and Stomach 31, *bi guan* or 'Thigh Gate'. Both these points form a kind of barrier. If the barrier is open, our energy (qi) can flow through the gate towards the ground. This allows us to ground ourselves. We can get things down to earth. However, tension and a lack of flexibility in this key zone indicate that we have lost the connection to our roots represented by our legs. And if a barrier is closed, traffic will back up. There will be stagnation and pressure, especially in the lower abdomen.

Legs

The strength of the stomach meridian is expressed in the state of the leg musculature. When there are sufficient supplies, both the centre and the periphery can be adequately nourished: strong thighs, strong lower legs. Or the opposite: if the stomach meridian is in a poor condition, there will be feeble and thin stilts which easily buckle under strain. The musculature along the tibia barely exists. Any deficiency in this area tends to be particularly apparent along the section of the meridian between the points Stomach 37, *shang ju xu* or 'Upper Great Void', and Stomach 39, *xia ju xu* or 'Lower Great Void'. Weakness in this part of the lower leg makes it difficult to run three miles further than anybody else. If you would like to bring more energy to this area, then Stomach 36, *zu san li* or 'Leg Three Miles', is the master point.

The Stomach Meridian: Key Points

- Associated element: Earth element
- Quality: Yang
- Time on the organ clock: 7am–9am
- Animal quality: Dragon
- Partner meridian: Large intestine meridian
- Twinned meridian: Spleen meridian
- Opposite meridian: Pericardium meridian

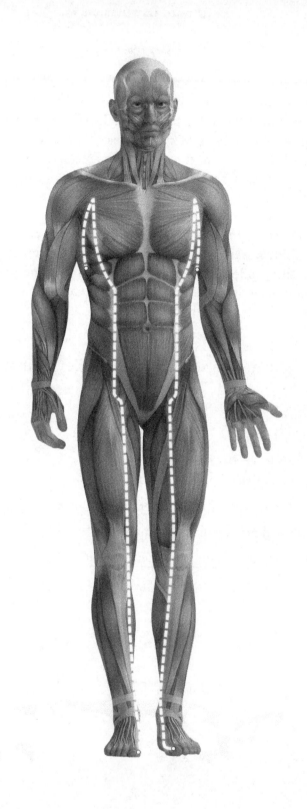

Chapter 6

The Spleen Meridian

The Primordial Mother and the Centre

Questions for the Spleen Meridian

- Am I able to give myself care, love and attention?
- Am I able to enjoy life? Am I able to make life pleasurable for myself?
- Do I let myself be thrown off balance easily?
- Do I easily get out of balance?
- Am I able to remain calm and stable in challenging situations?
- Am I able to give and share?
- Am I able to trust my gut feeling?
- Am I at home in my body?
- Am I able to deal with thoughts and feelings clearly and mindfully?

The Life Principle of the Spleen Meridian

We generally only talk about the middle when it has been lost. When it's not there any more, we long for it. The desire for a stable centre is like searching for the eye of the hurricane amidst the turbulences of life. It's like searching for a stable fulcrum to balance external and internal requirements. The desire to be centred is the desire for comfort and security. Our centre is our calm anchor, our most important reference point, where we can compose ourselves. It's a safe place to which we can return whenever we are looking for stability and peace. In our centre, nothing needs to happen, nothing needs to be attended to, nothing forces us into activity. In our centre, we can find true contentment. Preserving the strength of the centre is the life principle of the spleen meridian.

If you rest within yourself, you will have a clear yet relaxed connection to your identity and your body. You dwell in the centre of your own home. You are at home. Being at home is being present. Focus and awareness aren't scattered in the periphery of your personality but are concentrated in the core: I am. Without the need to be anything: I am. Without the need to have anything: I am. Without the need to do anything: I am. The deep-seated feeling of pleasant contentment with oneself is the hallmark of a strong spleen meridian.

In TCM, and in contrast to Western medicine, the spleen is one of the most important organs. It is an umbrella term for the entire digestive tract and the abdomen, which, indeed, represents the physical centre of our body. When the digestive tract works well, our body is excellently provided for: juicy flesh, strong blood. A well-nourished and tangible human being. The spleen is the primordial mother of our system. She's always present; there's always something on the table, and you're always given something to take home with you. However, not only does the spleen nourish our physical shell, but it also supplies the mind and the spirit. A well-developed spleen meridian allows us to be our own mother and to give ourselves what every mother feels towards her children: love, warmth and acceptance. The life principle of the spleen stands for unconditional self-love and self-pleasure. The spleen meridian sweetens our life. It is like a cosy kitchen that always welcomes us.

If we accept ourselves just as we are, if we love and enjoy ourselves, then we can also give without wanting or expecting anything in return. From the abundance of a strong centre arises the desire to contribute to the world with our abilities and gifts. True abundance wants to be shared and distributed because of the joy of giving, the joy of proliferating what is good and beautiful. Other people are not seen as competitors over whom we're trying to gain an advantage, but as allies on our journey through life, who have the same long-ings and desires as we do. They are seen as part of a big family whose load-bearing centre is the earth. There's enjoyable companionship and socialising. This, too, is an aspect of the life principle of the spleen: it likes giving. It likes people. It is gregarious. It appreciates togetherness.

However, genuine connections – whether relationships, friend-ships or work-related connections – are only possible when we are able to remain true to ourselves. This is where the true strength of our centre will manifest itself. If the life principle of the spleen isn't well evolved, the centre can become destabilised quite easily, even by minor challenges, and we quickly lose our balance. And if we don't manage to return to our centre, we might start looking for a replacement outside of ourselves. We turn other people or activities into our new centre. We're not at home in ourselves any more. Our own centre is missing something. To fill this hole, the spleen merid-ian often starts giving, but now it wants something in return – and not just anything. It craves the love and attention it can't supply itself. It thus turns into a mother who will do everything for her children in order to be seen and accepted by them. She sacrifices herself. She makes herself dependent. She turns into a never-tiring, somewhat intrusive, but ultimately helpless helper who is a long way from being centred in herself.

Within the first meridian family, the life principle of the spleen is the last one to develop. Preceded by the lung, large intestine and stomach meridians, it has an integrative character, transforming the features of the first three meridians into flesh and blood. The spleen makes things tangible. It channels into the centre. It consol-idates. Like a mother, facilitating peace and stability in her family.

The Spleen Meridian and the Body

The Hara and the Strength of the Centre

The Buddha combines many qualities that reflect the life principle of the spleen: presence, mindfulness, resting in one's centre, resting in oneself. The deep connection with one's own nature results, in turn, in a deep connection to other people, allowing compassion to arise and be expressed. The Buddha is the primordial mother for spiritual and emotional matters. It's for a good reason that the Buddha is often depicted with a big belly, much bigger than it could ever be in real life. Being so conspicuously rotund has nothing to do with decadence and a licentious tendency to opulent meals, but is rather an expression of the abundant energy and strength the Enlightened One has built up in his abdomen. Such abundance can be shared with those looking for support. The Buddha gives from his centre, which is referred to as *dantian* in China and *hara* in Japan. *Dantian* means 'cinnabar field'; *hara* means 'abdomen' but also 'source of life'.

The *hara* is the physical centre of gravity and plays a leading role in many Asian arts, but especially in martial arts, because a well-aligned body with a strong centre of gravity is not that easily pushed out of balance and returns more quickly to its centre when it has become imbalanced. This principle can also be applied to the psyche. If your mental centre of gravity is in the *hara*, your mind can achieve tremendous and unshakeable stability. This results in confident calmness and a deep inner peace. It is a question of focus. The psycho-emotional centre of gravity follows our attention: either our attention rests with equanimity in our centre, or it leaves its home and scatters, primarily in the external world. If the latter is the case, the spirit can easily lose its balance should the wind of life blow more harshly. We become a tree whose strength is not in its trunk but rests entirely in its branches. The result is instability without an anchor for rambling thoughts, roots for rising emotions or protective walls for fears and worries. It's easy to fall over – something that may well happen when the spleen energy is weak. For this reason, most meditation and yoga techniques explicitly aim at strengthening the *hara*. The centre is governed by clarity and stillness. It is the safe haven for our attention and our life force. It stands for the powerfully integrated life principle of the spleen.

However, our current times are quite challenging for this particular life principle. The natural belly has disappeared from our culture. We block out the replete fullness of a relaxed centre, and in doing so we commit hara-kiri to our wellbeing and our existence.

We prune and cut through our centre. With tight and constricting clothing. With sucking in our stomach. With the constant fight that advertising and the media force upon us, every single day and on all available channels: flat is good, fat is bad. Tension instead of relaxation. A six-pack instead of inner values. Youthful hyperactivity instead of compassion and benevolence. Illusion instead of reality. External form but inner emptiness. A fight with an acid flavour, as bitter as embittered.

The spleen, however, likes it sweet. It is the self-sufficient primordial mother with the best breast milk in the world, as sweet as love itself. Love is accepting. Self-love is self-acceptance. However, constantly succumbing to the feeling that we're not beautiful enough, good enough or clever enough will remove us from the sweetness of life. The primordial mother loves her children as they are, rather than as they should be. Accordingly, the spleen's crucial questions to the centre are: Am I able to accept myself as I am? Am I able to give love to myself? Am I able to sweeten my everyday life, my activities, my relationships? If not, the sweetness missing in the spleen meridian will be compensated for with sweet foods. Sugar: nourishment for the starving soul. We try to fill up the lost centre with an excess of sweets but end up losing it even more. The *hara* gets bloated, becomes soft, spongy flab instead of energised fullness. Voluminous rubber rings, even obesity, to prevent drowning in the river of life. The disease: sugar addiction. Sugar disease: diabetes. It's for a reason that diabetes is on a global triumphal march. TCM considers diabetes a weakness of the spleen. We go belly-up. On all levels.

And that's because when we lose the *hara*, we also lose our inner stability, our home, our gut feeling. We're all at sea. We're not resting within ourselves. We're a bit lost. What helps is relaxation. By relaxing, we can feel more grounded. If we're more grounded, we can be more relaxed. Energy isn't wasted on getting unnecessary recognition or hunting for superficial attention. The energy thus saved can gather. It can gather in the source of life, in the *hara*, which can then become an expression of inner fulfilment. If well integrated, the life principle of the spleen stands for an energetically plump stomach; for a strong and stable centre.

Flatulence, a sensation of pressure in the abdomen, digestive disorders, being overweight, being underweight, diabetes, metabolic disorders, fatty liver, psychic instability...

Tissue and the Firmness of Being

The strength of the centre is a stabilising strength. If the life principle of the spleen, and therefore the cohesive quality of the centre, is only poorly developed, the periphery loses firmness. It begins to dissolve. This becomes particularly apparent in the texture of the connective and muscular tissue. As the name implies, the connective tissue binds the body and the organs together. The life principle of the spleen is a synonym for the entire digestive tract. It supplies and nourishes our body, and therefore also the tissue. When it is in good condition, tissue is taut, full of vitality and responsive. Ideally like that of a small child: firm, hearty and bursting with energy.

And then there's the opposite case: weak connective tissue. Flaccid and watery tissue that can't keep its form and texture, so that the entire body is out of shape. What was once a powerful supportive net has become soft. The body – our house – is disintegrating. The walls are dented and damp. They are losing their colour, and the plaster is coming off. Instability. Flooding. The result is pale, pasty and somewhat puffy skin. There are varicose veins due to the blood vessels losing their integrity. Loose stools, often with undigested food, because the digestive tract is lacking the strength and tone to sufficiently process the bolus. And there's also cellulite as well as oedema, and stretch marks. The tissue is easily malleable and sensitive, and bruises quickly when touched. The discoloured skin reflects how easy it is to leave an impression on people with a deficient spleen meridian. Weak tissue can be shaped without much effort. It's easy to put a mark on it. The same is true for the psyche. People who aren't firmly resting in their centre are susceptible to all kinds of influences. It's easy to groom them and to put a mark on them.

A spleen meridian with a poorly developed life principle can also have the effect that it is not only the body but also the spirit that becomes deformed without much resistance. But back to the *hara*: an uninhabited centre is like an uninhabited house. Either may be attractive to squatters. And weak tissue finds it difficult to hold out against that. It has lost its reactivity. Poor tone, poor resistance. People with a weak spleen meridian are quick to adopt the opinions of others since they lack a stable personality. They tend to conform. They are quick to let themselves be impressed. And if there is too much pressure, they are quick to break down. Deep fatigue spreads through their body, mentally, emotionally and physically.

What to do? Fight tooth and nail? Run away? That may be difficult since the muscles are tissue, too. According to TCM, the spleen nourishes the flesh and the limbs. What does that mean? It means first things first. First and foremost, the body requires energy for the central areas since the organs need to be well supplied. They are essential for survival. Only if there is a surplus of energy can this be transferred to the periphery. A strong spleen meridian is able to supply not only the centre but also the arms and legs with vigorous and nourishing energy, clearly visible in well-defined muscles. Strong calves. Strong forearms. Robust and healthy all round.

The spleen meridian is responsible for the upward direction of energy. If it is weak, the musculature, also being tissue, loses its tone and becomes weak, soft and sluggish, and increasingly gives in to gravity. It collapses. Knock knees, flat feet. You're glued to the ground and each step is an effort. A progressive weakness of the spleen meridian can even lead to organ prolapses. Nothing stays properly in its place any more. This is a far cry from how a healthy spleen meridian manifests: centredness, abundance, strength.

SYMPTOMS ASSOCIATED WITH THE SPLEEN MERIDIAN

Weak connective tissue, varicose veins, oedema, cellulite, prone to bruising easily, loose stools, watery diarrhoea, organ prolapses, fatigue, flat feet, knock knees...

The Spleen Meridian and the Psyche

Giving, Sharing and Dependency

For a person to be a nourishing mother to themselves requires a spleen with a well-developed and well-integrated life principle. This provides independence and self-sufficiency, especially emotionally. If you love and accept yourself, you don't need anybody doing this for you externally. You're able to create and maintain inner fullness yourself. This is the foundation for giving and sharing freely. Because giving and sharing should always come from a state of surplus: only then will nothing be expected in return. A strong spleen results in honest altruism. We are sufficiently centred and therefore we don't lose ourselves in the act of giving. And for this very reason we don't have to give it centre stage.

A weakened life principle of the spleen also likes to share, albeit with a different motivation. It gives in order to get recognition. It gives with the intention of getting something back. This is not giving freely; it is rather a deal, driven by the inner need for affection and attention. It is a form of longing, whose roots can often be found in early life experiences. Meridians are life principles that evolve. Often, it is about a disappointment or a rejection by the parents during childhood. If we have never felt, been given or experienced and witnessed love and validation, this will gnaw away at our feelings of self-worth. And impaired self-worth leads to insecurity. In such a scenario, it's difficult to rest firmly in our centre because this has to be built up in the first place. The result is a spleen meridian that is incapable of fully evolving. It can't offer support and stability. Others are therefore needed to fill that gap. There's also a desire to be needed. These are people who help in order to be helped. For them, helping becomes an obsession, an addiction, even a self-sacrifice.

A weakness in the life principle of the spleen meridian may have the effect that the need to validate ourselves through constant giving leads us to neglect our own desires, goals and boundaries. We cling to the people from whom, through constant, even meddlesome offers of assistance, we are desperately trying to wring at least an ounce of recognition. We make others the centre of our life. We turn other people into the centre we are lacking. The value we attribute to ourselves becomes dependent on others. We become dependent. We overburden ourselves until there's a complete deficiency of blood. In TCM, the spleen meridian is, among other things, responsible for the formation of blood. Blood supplies the entire body: the lifeblood of our bodies. And we will lose this lifeblood if we constantly allow others to suck us dry. What remains is the burnt-out helpless helper. Self-sacrifice in the role of the martyr.

But woe betide us if nothing comes back in return! Then the blood can quickly boil. Inside, there is a bubbling volcano that feels neither understood nor heard. Yet on the outside, the smile is maintained. Despite everything, we want to conform and be nice. The steam is vented only behind closed doors. We appear serene, even if we're close to burning up inside. What helps is keeping calm.

The desire to share and to help is a human trait as beautiful as it is deep. But a well has to be full if we want to scoop water out of it. A well-developed life principle of the spleen knows this. Every airline knows this: in case of a lack of oxygen, place the mask first over your own nose and mouth before assisting others. Otherwise, you may have trouble breathing and be unable to help anyone else, and ultimately others may have to look after you. Therefore it's so important to be a loving and mindful mother to yourself. This will lead you to inner abundance and contentment. It will lead you to independence. And then you can share and help generously.

Mindfulness and Circular Thinking

When you are grounded in yourself, you are at home, centred, present. The centre is clear and still – the eye of the hurricane. But when you leave this calm centre, the whirlwind of everyday life may catch up with you, and affect, in particular, your ability to think in an action- and goal-oriented way. Thoughts are like water, a continuous and never-ending river. By being focussed and mindful, we can guide and direct this river, supported by a well-developed spleen meridian. However, if we're unable to do this, we tend to get carried away by the stream of our thoughts, again and again. Indeed, we are overwhelmed by the stream of our thoughts and can't control the flow. We ruminate around the clock. We're caught on the merry-go-round of thinking.

Ruminating creates problems in the head that in reality don't even exist. You ruminate about this and that, about others, about yourself, about a thousand things. You ruminate for rumination's sake, without wasting a single thought on an actual solution. It's all about: Why? Why? Why, oh why? Although the stomach meridian, the spleen's partner meridian, is equally susceptible to never-ending mind games, it doesn't ask for the why, but for the how. The thinking of the stomach is selective; the thinking of the spleen spreads out. Just as a weak spleen meridian is incapable of holding together the tissue, so it is unable to give structure and form to thoughts. In the long run, this requires a lot of energy – after all, the brain has to work flat out without finding a solution. Rumination blocks the view to any course of action. Rumination can lead to indecision and procrastination. This, in turn, can trigger feelings of powerlessness, sadness or anger. That's because you're not progressing. You're treading water. And what about your self-esteem? In this kind of scenario, it won't be particularly well nourished. Rumination is often the substrate for depression and helplessness. The corresponding character profile is the classic victim role, wallowing in passivity and neediness.

Rumination is a characteristic trait of a spleen with a deficient life principle. One thing is clear: rumination leads nowhere, other than away from one's centre. And the only way out of the cul-de-sac of rumination is the path back to the centre, the path of mindfulness. When you're mindful, there's no time for rumination. Mindfulness is the most effective opposition to 'would've, could've, should've'. Mindfulness takes us into the present moment. Mindfulness is an acute observer. Mindfulness can interrupt the stream of thoughts. Mindfulness considers thoughts to be like a river and decides whether it wants to go for a swim or not. Mindfulness is centredness. Mindfulness is the expression of a strong spleen. It allows us to have a calm yet alert mind that isn't easily distracted or shaken. And that brings us back to the Buddha with his thick belly, his stable centre of gravity, as the archetype of a well-developed life principle of the spleen meridian. Thus endowed, one can wholeheartedly immerse oneself in the present moment, in activities, in other human beings, without losing oneself.

Signs of an Imbalanced and Balanced Spleen Meridian

Signs of an Imbalanced Spleen Meridian

- Weak tissue, tendency to loose stools, water accumulations
- Difficulty concentrating, being distracted
- Tiredness, heavy limbs, blood deficiency
- Tendency to low or depressive moods
- Tendency to being overweight, metabolic disorders, diabetes
- Constant rumination, emotionally and mentally unstable

Signs of a Balanced Spleen Meridian

- Powerful and well-nourished body, firm tissue
- Good body awareness, good gut feeling
- Emotionally and mentally centred and stable
- Mindful and aware demeanour, clarity of thought
- Self-love, self-acceptance, self-contentedness
- Highly sociable, socially competent
- Capacity for giving, supporting and caring for others

How to Strengthen the Life Principle of the Spleen Meridian

Cultivating Self-love

Once a week, take the time for a date with yourself. Plan it carefully. Put yourself in the shoes of another person: What would they have to do to truly win you over? What day and time do you favour? What do you enjoy doing? What is the best way for someone to communicate to you their appreciation of and affection towards you? Organise this date with the same effort, attention and joyful anticipation a person who loves you would invest. Dress accordingly.

Ensure the atmosphere is right. Give yourself the gift of attention and kindness. Spoil yourself. Simply do it. Enjoy it.

Meditation

Meditation is the best way to build up one's centre as a stable anchor for body, mind and spirit. Think of the Buddha. Simply sit down. Bring your attention to your belly and use it as a focal point to which you can return again and again when your mind begins to wander. This will happen, and very often, too. Simply bring your attention back to your centre, kindly and gently. Meditation should be a daily routine. Morning is the best time to lay a mindful foundation for the day and collect yourself before embarking on the turbulences of everyday life. At first, five minutes will suffice. In order to progress with your meditation practice, continuity is much more important than duration.

The Pathway of the Spleen Meridian

The spleen meridian begins at Spleen 1 at the inner corner of the big toe. It then courses laterally along the big toe, at the border of the dorsal and plantar aspects and traverses the palpable and visible base joint of the big toe. Just distal and proximal to this joint are the important points Spleen 2 and Spleen 3 respectively. From there, the spleen meridian follows the first metatarsal bone, again along the border of the dorsal and plantar aspects to a point in a depression on the anterior inferior border of the medial malleolus: Spleen 5.

The spleen meridian travels further along the anterior border of the medial malleolus to ascend the inner border of the tibia, where Spleen 6 can be found three thumb-widths directly above the medial malleolus. The spleen meridian now continues along the inner border of the tibia to Spleen 9, located in a depression on the lower border of the medial epicondyle of the tibia. From Spleen 9, the meridian curves towards the medial border of the kneecap (patella), following this border upwards to Spleen 10, situated two thumb-widths above the upper and medial patellar corner. It ascends further in the anatomical groove between two heads (rectus femoris, vastus medialis) of the four-headed quadriceps. The meridian follows this groove, but once it has reached the last third of the thigh, where the sartorius crosses the quadriceps, it begins to turn more laterally to reach Spleen 12, three and a half thumb-widths lateral to the anterior midline and level with the upper border of the pubic symphysis.

From Spleen 12, the spleen meridian veers even further laterally to Spleen 13, located 0.7 thumb-widths above Spleen 12 and four thumb-widths lateral to the midline. It then ascends in a straight line, four thumb-widths lateral to the anterior midline, until it reaches the lower border of the ribcage. Spleen 16 can be found one and a half thumb-widths below the cartilage of the ninth rib. From there, the spleen meridian curves diagonally in a lateral direction, along the border between the anterior and lateral chest. The next landmark is Spleen 17, located in the fifth intercostal space, six thumb-widths lateral to the midline.

The spleen meridian remains at this distance to the midline as it ascends to Spleen 20, which can be found in the second intercostal space, directly vertically below Lung 1. At Spleen 20, the spleen meridian turns around and courses to the final point of the meridian, Spleen 21, located on the mid-axillary line in the sixth intercostal space.

Key Areas of the Spleen Meridian

Feet and Legs

Our feet and legs reflect how we stand in life. The question to ask the spleen is whether we are stable and strong enough to be able to stand up for ourselves. The spleen meridian, as expressed by its pathway, governs the inside of the legs. When the spleen meridian is weak, this area can collapse. Everything is soft and without strength: the tissue and the muscles, the entire musculoskeletal structure, as well as the blood vessels. Instead of being carried, we crumple. Varicose veins and knock knees are therefore typical features of a weakness in the spleen meridian. The knees are lacking stability around the location of Spleen 9, 'Yin Mound Spring' or *yin ling quan.* In TCM, the quality of yin has a preserving, nourishing strength. Without this strength, everything dissolves and the spring on the Yin Mound overflows. When the spleen is weak, we therefore often find water accumulations or swellings in the general area of the knee. Chronic degenerative wear and tear of the inner meniscus is considered a spleen disorder: the cartilage dissolves as it hasn't been sufficiently nourished by the spleen.

The missing structural support of the spleen can also manifest at the ankles: in cases of spleen deficiency, the ankles are prone to buckling inwards. Slightly superior to the ankle is the point Spleen 6, the 'Meeting Point of the Three Yin' or *san yin jiao.* It is a good diagnostic point for gauging the state of the body's yin. Soft tissue or water accumulations around this point may be a sign that the spleen has lost its firmness.

This state can be particularly clearly pronounced around the point Spleen 4, 'Grandfather Grandson' or *gong sun,* located on the inside of the arch of the foot. Ideally, we stand actively in the here and now, between the past and the future. Between grandfather and grandson. Precisely in the centre. Our centre. We can move freely, learn from the past and march confidently into the future. However, when the spleen is weak, our feet will be flat. When standing, the entire sole of the foot comes to rest on the ground. We stick to the ground, and along with the arch of the foot, we have lost any bounce and jumping ability. Sluggishness and heaviness set in. Walking is a cause of bother, especially since a hallux valgus is a further common symptom of spleen deficiency. It pulls the big toe medially as the spleen meridian is unable to put up any resistance. And this occurs precisely at the location of one of its most important points: Spleen 3, 'Supreme White' or *tai bai.* When the spleen is strong, we can climb the highest mountains with it, to where the glaciers kiss heaven.

Hara

The *hara* – the abdomen – is the key area of the spleen meridian. Many acupuncture points indicate its importance. Directly in the navel is the point Ren Mai 8, 'Spirit Palace' or *shen que.* This is precisely the area that should be the home of our mind, our focus

— the centre of the centre. Right in the middle. Slightly below Ren Mai 8 are the points Ren Mai 4 and Ren Mai 6. Ren Mai 4 is the 'Origin Pass' or *guan yuan*; Ren Mai 6, the 'Sea of Qi' or *qi hai*. If our consciousness is rooted deeply in the *hara*, then we can return to our origin; we can connect with the core of our being as if entering through a gate. This gives us strength and energy, manifesting in the Sea of Qi, the sea of energy.

Conversely, problems can arise if we have a tense relationship with our centre. Then we may have a knot in our stomach, something that can be clearly felt at Spleen 14, 'Abdomen Knot' or *fu jie*, or at Spleen 16, 'Abdomen Sorrow' or *fu ai*. Both these points are also located near the navel.

The Spleen Meridian: Key Points

- Associated element: Earth element

- Quality: Yin

- Time on the organ clock: 9am–11am

- Animal quality: Snake

- Partner meridian: Stomach meridian

- Twinned meridian: Lung meridian

- Opposite meridian: Triple heater meridian

Chapter 7

The First Meridian Family: Lungs, Large Intestine, Stomach and Spleen

Basic Provisions

In TCM, every organ is allocated a two-hour time slot during the course of the day when it is particularly active and supplied with additional energy. This energy cycle begins with the lungs. Their excess time begins at 3am and lasts until 5am, the time when the day begins, the time of new beginnings. The lung is followed by the large intestine (5am to 7am), the stomach (7am to 9am), and finally the spleen (9am to 11am). In short, we get up yawning (lungs), go to the toilet (large intestine), have our breakfast (stomach) and digest (spleen). Of course, this programme is usually compressed due to the demands of reality. In Asia, however, gentle exercises for strengthening and maintaining health are practised predominantly during lung time. And even in the West, it is generally accepted that exercising before breakfast stimulates the cardiovascular system and has a beneficial effect on the entire day. A bowel movement in the morning is considered equally important.

Whichever way we start the day, these four meridians are connected; they represent the first quarter of the big energy cycle. They represent the first meridian family, and each meridian family has a core theme to which all meridians contribute their respective life principle for the benefit of a bigger and well-functioning whole. Accordingly, the central questions of the first meridian family are: Am I able to provide for myself? Am I able to feed myself?

These questions refer to all levels, their material, mental and emotional aspects. The focus of the first meridian family corresponds to the first three levels of Maslow's pyramid of needs.

On an even more fundamental level, these four meridians enable us to live and survive in general. In order to define an independent living being as such, we first need a boundary. On a cellular level, this is the cell membrane. No membrane, no cell. The lung meridian takes care of this initial boundary. However, a boundary should not be too impermeable. To safeguard life, there has to be an exchange. The lungs facilitate opening the boundary. And, of course, cells need energy. This is supplied by the stomach meridian. It provides and processes what is needed. Further processing, as well as providing the necessary energy, is, in turn, the task of the spleen meridian. The large intestine meridian, finally, deals with the elimination of waste. The first meridian family is truly an entity fit for survival.

Its four meridians develop immediately after birth; they are the first to come into their own. Independent life, separate from the mother's direct supplies, begins with the lung meridian and the first breath. From then on, the infant has to rely on its own energy supplies, which have to be safeguarded at all times. The large intestine meridian is also active quite quickly to eliminate the meconium. The discharge of this first tangible metabolic end product often occurs during the first day and is a sign that all is well with the baby's digestive tract. The stomach meridian, in turn, ensures that the infant's hungry mouth instinctively finds the mother's breast, and that it is able to suckle and swallow. And last but not least, the spleen comes into play in order to process what has been ingested, transforming it into flesh and blood; this too has to be learned.

It can take time – weeks and even months – for the digestive tract to function more or less well. What has been taken in won't stay there. There is belching and vomiting. Then there is bloating, constipation and diarrhoea – in sum, a colourful and constantly changing mix. The spleen meridian also needs time before it can fully come into its own. Parents can tell you a thing or two about this. In the first phase of life, everything is about the most basic needs. The infant's brain is preconditioned with only a few behavioural patterns relevant from an evolutionary point of view, which can all be assigned to the first meridian family. They are about breathing, eating, sleeping, eliminating. But they're also about security, safety, affection and love. A baby requires emotional nourishment, too; it needs nourishment for the soul. Touch is another crucial factor. Touch is mediated through skin contact, and the skin is assigned to the lung meridian. Touch is direct nourishment for the life principle of the lung meridian. Touch nourishes the 'yes' to life. Children are born with an innate need for attachment. This is an important key for survival since only a reliable caregiver can safeguard the child's existence. Attachment is reinforced through bodily and emotional closeness creating trust. Basic trust for the 'yes' to life.

A lack of touch can impair physical, emotional and mental development. This is also true for the development of the meridians. They are like plants. Under optimal conditions, plants thrive, take up their predetermined space and go about their tasks and functions smoothly. But if the development of the meridians is impaired or conditions for their development are suboptimal, they are unable to fully evolve their life principles and a deficit will ensue. This can result in weak points that may remain with us for our entire life. Disharmonies in the first meridian family often have to do with the feeling of not getting enough, being undersupplied in important areas of our lives or not having the strength to get from life what would make us happy and content. For a baby that was never emotionally nourished, perhaps because it was unwanted, the feeling of being unloved can develop into a driving force during adulthood, resulting in a wide range of compensatory behaviours. When our intuitive sense of boundaries is missing, perhaps because we were not touched enough so that we were never able to truly feel and experience ourselves, we can turn into risk takers in later life, requiring intense stimuli and adventures as we seek confirmation of our identity. Early deficits don't always have to result in severe problems affecting the quality of life, but the substrate certainly exists. It is a given that there can't be a dynamic and fruitful balance when in a four-spoke wheel, three of the spokes are too loose and one is too tight. Such a wheel is certain not to run smoothly.

Each meridian family has a loose connection to our personal developmental history, with the first meridian family evolving most strongly during the first six to twelve months. When teething begins and the child starts to move around the room, the foundations for the first meridian family have been laid. Up to that point everything revolves around the front of the body, which is dominated by the meridians of the lungs, large intestine, stomach and spleen. The change from one meridian family to the next is a smooth transition that depends on many individual factors. When one meridian family has not sufficiently matured, this will affect the subsequent development. Imagine a house. The first meridian family is the foundation. Sooner or later, unstable foundations will become obvious in all further storeys. For this reason, it's important to check the foundations now and again, even if disorders or problems manifest in other meridians. After all, it's for a good reason that the first meridian family takes first place in the organ clock and the energy cycle. It can only pass on what it is able to give. It's up to us to create a satisfactory surplus – by developing the life principles of its meridians.

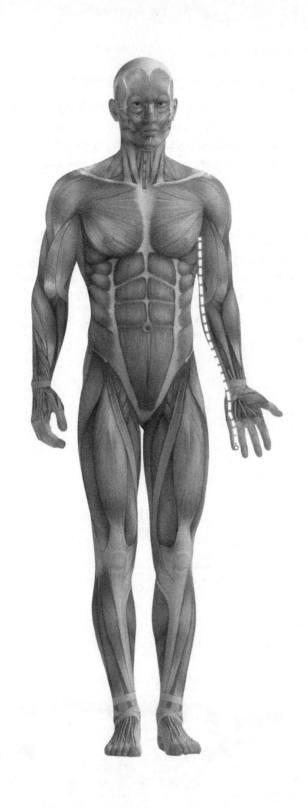

Chapter 8

The Heart Meridian

The Compassionate Emperor

Questions for the Heart Meridian

- Do I get enthusiastic easily?
- Am I able to be compassionate and eager?
- Am I able to inspire myself as well as others?
- Do I get interested in things easily?
- Am I able to communicate well?
- Am I able to express myself clearly and distinctly?
- Do I find it easy to address and voice any relevant matters?
- Do I get emotional easily?
- Am I easily thrown off balance by feelings?
- Am I often absent-minded and forgetful?
- Am I easily distracted?
- Do I find it difficult to stay focussed for a long period of time?
- Do I get nervous easily?
- Do I start to sweat quickly when I am stressed?
- Is my sleep deep and restorative?

The Life Principle of the Heart Meridian

In TCM, the heart is considered the emperor of the organs. In Western medicine, the heart is at the top of the organ hierarchy as well: it is the engine of the body. It keeps the system going, and it nourishes and supports all other organs via the blood. When the heart is well, all is well. Without a strong emperor, the empire will disintegrate. TCM further expands the already existential role of the heart, which is not only the foundation of our life but also the basis for consciously experiencing life. The heart is the home of our spirit, which in TCM is referred to as *shen*. The *shen* is the seat of our perception. It is the authority without which a self-experiential 'I' wouldn't even exist. The *shen* is the emperor who governs and guides. All other meridians are subordinate to him. In TCM, the function of the *shen* is as pivotal as that of the brain in biomedicine.

Without *shen*, our body would be not much more than a functional shell that, based on purely instinctive impulses and actions, rattles off its plan in a more or less satisfying manner. Only the *shen* endows us with a heart and soul. It invigorates us. It represents our capacity for enthusiasm. It ensures that we organise our life in a hearty, lionhearted and heartfelt way. A well-developed life principle of the heart meridian shines in cheerful passion, unbridled enthusiasm and ceaseless inspiration. This has a profound influence on our entire body. When the boss is in a good mood, so will be the staff. When the heart is well, so will be the other organs. No other meridian has the capacity to supply us with energy as quickly as the heart meridian. No matter how healthy our diet, how much we exercise, whether we meditate, practise yoga or deal with our personal development daily and consistently, if the heart doesn't support our efforts, they won't make much of a difference. With a listless emperor, our *joie de vivre* quickly goes to pieces, and, sooner or later, our health as well.

It is the mandate of the heart meridian that we dedicate ourselves to activities or people with all our heart, with joy and commitment. Only in this way can our heart be open. Only in this way can our heart be light, and our inner sun begin to shine. This is tangible, it is visible. Because the *shen* is mirrored in the eyes. Eyes can shine, laugh, sparkle. An alert and lively look, expressing *joie de vivre* and clarity. An unclouded perception is a further expression of a well-developed heart meridian. As the meridian of the fire element, the heart meridian brings light into the darkness. The heart meridian can see, both externally and internally. And only those who can see with their hearts can see properly, deeply and penetratingly. A strong heart meridian allows us insights into life, into ourselves and, ideally, into the true nature of being. It is this insight that subsequently leads to clarity. Clarity of the spirit, clarity of the soul. And clarity of language, since, as the German adage has it, we carry our heart on our tongue (and not on our sleeve), and our ability to express ourselves clearly and distinctly is also associated with the heart meridian.

But, of course, when talking about the heart meridian, we also need to talk about love. Love has many faces. And the heart meridian knows them all, from the all-consuming fire of passion to spiritual love. The ability to open up our heart rises and falls with the development of the heart meridian. On one end of the scale is the heart of stone, sulky, lonely and morose. The soul loses its warmth. The emperor loses his power, and so does the entire system. Just how strong the influence of the heart meridian can become is most obvious during times of lovesickness, when the world seems to lose all its colour and meaning.

If the life principle of the heart meridian is only poorly developed, this can lead to an underlying depressed mood. The inner fire has gone out. A well-developed life principle of the heart meridian, on the other hand, finds it easy to fall in love again and again, preferably daily, ideally with life itself. The pulse of the heart resonates with the pulse of existence.

The Heart Meridian and the Body

Face, Eyes and Tongue

The face can be seen as a direct mirror of the heart energy. The expression of the heart meridian is particularly dense in two areas: the eyes and the tongue. While many meridians connect with the eyes, none is expressed as directly as the heart meridian: the eyes are the windows of the soul, they are the gate to our consciousness, they are the headlights of the *shen*. The eyes are the most honest part of the face. However hard you may try to keep your countenance or your poker face, a look says more than a thousand words. No other part of the body can mediate such a wide range of emotions as the eyes. This is due to the special role of the heart as the emperor of the organs. The emperor is in direct contact with all organs; he knows what shape his country is in. He's empathic, he's compassionate, he shares joy. He keeps an eye on everybody. And everybody is keeping an eye on him. Whether it's fear, grief, joy, mistrust, contentment or anger – everything is reflected in the eyes, as is the emperor's character. Eyes can be kind, hard, gentle, powerful, enthusiastic or absent. And sometimes they can appear as if someone is completely out of their mind.

A strongly developed heart energy stands for the ability to see and understand things clearly. Ideally, there should be hardly any or no scales at all on the eyes that might blur the view of oneself and of life. You walk through life with your eyes wide open. You like to make eye contact because your heart is open. You are looking for and enjoying connections with others. You are outgoing and sociable. Your demeanour can make people feel uncomfortable because it can seem as if you are able to look through them. Pure vision, pure heart, pure mirror: we can see and recognise ourselves in the person opposite. If that feels unpleasant, some introspection may be of benefit since people with a poorly developed life principle of the heart meridian are often blind to their own issues.

Sometimes, however, introspection can become exaggerated. You may get overly familiar with your inner world while ignoring the reality on your doorstep and shying away from confronting it. The emperor is introverted and scared of going out into the street. He deals primarily with his own issues. Hiding in his shell is what he loves best. The heart is withdrawn and not very sociable; perhaps there are even underlying autistic traits. The eyes tend to be vacant and insecure: no radiance, no luminosity, an inward gaze. It feels as if people like that aren't really present, as if they don't really participate in life. No trace of enthusiasm, no hint of passion. What's missing is perspective, the ability to look ahead. The key to resolving this is confidence and courage. Be lionhearted and open up.

Conversely, if the spirit has a tendency to happily wander about in the wide blue yonder, it has to be asked to return a bit closer to home. This, too, can be a problem of the heart meridian: an excessive outward orientation. A form of extraversion that serves as protection. Such people like to keep busy with all kinds of things except for themselves. Looking into the distance, foresight, long-sightedness: while this obviously provides an insight into many exotic realms, their homeland is a blank page, including everything that may be going on there – from suppressed problems to dormant potentials. This is a kind of tunnel vision. Such people don't want to look too closely or too deeply. They prefer frivolity and lightness. They like to be evasive and to go off on tangents; there is always distraction. This restlessness can be recognised in their eyes – nervousness, constant motion, quasi-protruding eyes.

And then there are dull eyes indicating another suboptimal state of the *shen*. Since our consciousness loves clarity, looking through blurry eyes is like looking through fog. As a result, our perception becomes equally hazy: confusion instead of focus, fuzziness instead of acuity. Out of sight, out of mind. An emperor who is a bit lost and far from being present.

A heart meridian with a healthy life principle facilitates intro-spection as well as panoramic vision. The emperor knows perfectly well what's going on in the basement of his palace and at the borders of his empire. He has the overview and very few blind spots. This allows him to respond appropriately. Furthermore, a lively heart energy allows quick changes in perspective; it allows us to see things with different eyes, to consider a situation from a different angle. A lively heart energy also stands for astuteness and mental flexibility.

The eyes express so much about the emperor's character. The same is true of the tongue, as this is where, according to a German proverb, we carry our heart; a branch of the heart meridian does, indeed, terminate at the tip of the tongue. Our ability to commu-nicate is connected directly to the state of the heart meridian. Communication connects. Communication builds bridges between humans. Communication is a means to express consciousness. A well-developed life principle of the heart meridian reveals itself in clear, lively and beautiful speech which directly mirrors the spirit's clarity, openness, freedom and vitality. The voice is carried by pres-ence and alertness. We need a healthy heart meridian to express and communicate what is close to our heart. A strong emperor is able to be transparent in all aspects and circumstances. He says what needs to be said; he's direct and authentic.

Conversely, a poorly developed life principle of the heart can have the effect that you would rather bite your tongue than say something, however much it may be on the tip of your tongue, even if it makes your tongue burn. Instead of giving words free rein, they are curbed. People with weak heart energy talk little and reluctantly; they speak with a heavy tongue, indistinct words and soporific monotony. They hate and avoid communication, and they get palpitations if they have to be the centre of attention and say something. They find it difficult to convey how they feel. However, they are precisely the kind of people for whom it would be so important to express themselves regularly because what isn't expressed builds up inner pressure, and inner pressure constricts the heart. At the bottom of the inability for open and lively communication is often insecurity and fear, just as a shock can literally leave someone utterly speechless. It's for a good reason that a meaningful conversation allowing us to get everything off our chest can have such a healing effect. For the life principle of our heart, it's important to pour out our heart regularly to get rid of the pressure holding it down. This is liberating; it clarifies. Clarification leads to clarity, and clarity benefits the heart.

A lack of clarity, on the other hand, can cause people to speak duplicitously with a forked tongue. An imbalanced heart meridian often results in a distorted perception of reality since consciousness becomes clouded. And consciousness that is unstable and not anchored is like a flame, jumping frantically around, resting here, resting there. You never know where you stand. In small children, the heart meridian is often still fragile. One moment they say 'no', the next moment 'yes', and each time they do so with utter conviction. Imagination can become reality and vice versa. This is not about lying; rather, it's about what they perceive. It can happen in adults, too. It makes them hard to grasp, and it's even harder to build up trust in them. But if we can see this behaviour as an imbalance of the heart energy, it makes it easier to accept.

Disorders concerning language acquisition and development are also connected with the life principle of the heart meridian, including impaired speech comprehension, limited vocabulary, difficulty articulating and insecurity about applying correct grammar. In this context, too, there is a close connection with the *shen*. In TCM, the brain and the heart belong together, and therefore the capacity for mental processing is considered to pertain to the heart in the wider sense, especially with regard to reason, comprehension and difficulties in understanding. For this reason, the heart meridian is used to treat many speech disorders.

A harmonious heart meridian supports luminous eyes, clear communication and a lively expression. It brings radiance to the face. One can see that the emperor is well.

SYMPTOMS ASSOCIATED WITH THE HEART MERIDIAN

Any type of visual disorders, exaggerated extroverted or introverted behaviour, confusion, ambiguity, indistinct or mumbled speech, stammering, delayed speech development, language loss...

A Question of Blood

According to TCM, the heart, as the emperor of the organs, mediates its orders by means of the blood. The blood allows the emperor to reach even the most remote corners of his empire. The heart requires the blood to be calm, so that it can go about its task without friction. The heart is by far the most sensitive organ; it is the most easily hurt, the most easily touched, the most easily moved, especially by emotions. Whatever their nature, whether positive or negative, whether they are coming our way externally or are arising due to our own reactions, emotions influence both blood and heart quickly and directly. Fear can make the blood freeze in our veins. Resentment can stir up the blood or even make it boil. Joy can make the heart sing; it can make our heart feel as though it is about to burst. Effusive excitement or arousal will make it flutter. But what jumps and flutters can easily stumble or lose its rhythm. This should not happen, either to the emperor or to the heart. The emperor is the boss. He has to keep his sangfroid.

The hallmarks of a well-developed life principle of the heart meridian are great emotional and psychological stability, as well as the ability to remain clear and focussed even in difficult situations. The heart blood has to be envisioned as the coolant in an engine. If it functions flawlessly, you can accelerate without any risk. But too little coolant and the engine will start to overheat with the slightest strain. A weakness in the heart meridian responds to even the most minute stimuli: we're either on top of the world or in the depths of despair. We easily run hot, so that we are constantly restless and tense with an increased tendency to hyperactivity. Even minor challenges lead to shaking and sweating, particularly in the area of the heart meridian's origin: the armpits. This results in people being unstable and distracted by the most trivial details. They have the attention span of a small child. Communication with such people is difficult to follow since they have the tendency to speak very fast and constantly lose their thread. Not even at night is there any rest for the sensitive emperor: his sleep tends to be very light, restless and disturbed by vivid dreaming. This gnaws away at his psyche, which becomes more and more unstable. It can lead to an increased startle response including panic attacks.

In its advanced stage, a weak heart meridian causes the emperor increasingly to lose his focus. He gets confused, forgetful and absent-minded. His perception is distorted, and the boundary between reality and imagination may become blurred. In the worst case, the *shen* simply looks for another home; it disappears in a dreamworld or anchors itself in another personality. Be it mania or schizophrenia, TCM considers many mental illnesses to have their root in the heart meridian. Conversely, by strengthening the heart meridian, the psyche can find stillness and health. What the heart deserves is a calm *shen*, steadiness, clarity and mindful awareness.

SYMPTOMS ASSOCIATED WITH THE HEART MERIDIAN

Emotional and mental instability, inner restlessness, tension, hyper-activity, fluttering about, arrhythmias, sleep disorders, confusion, forgetfulness, being very easily startled, manic behaviour...

The Heart Meridian and the Psyche

Inspiration, Creativity and Enthusiasm

Inspiration and creativity represent the essence of the life principle of the heart meridian. The word 'inspiration' derives from the Latin *inspiratio,* which can be translated as 'ensoulment' or 'breathing in'. What the heart meridian breathes in is the 'spiritus', the spirit, which 'inspires'. Inspiration and creativity allow us to organise our existence independently, autonomously and freely. The emperor governs according to his own beliefs and ideas; he is accountable to no one. He neither buckles nor bends. He does as he pleases; he does what he really likes to do, and he acts in order to follow his destiny. The heart is an exuberant creator who passionately stands in the midst of life and creates its own reality. The heart is at the heart of strong personalities who are little impressed by conventions and popular ideas.

A well-developed life principle of the heart meridian manifests in heightened joy, in enthusiastic commitment and an exceptionally intense interest in all kinds of subject matters, activities and people. People with such a heart meridian are often in a state of effusive excitement that gives them strength and great stamina. Inspiration and enthusiasm are the life elixir par excellence and the strongest source of energy we can draw on. They electrify us with their never-waning stimuli. They let our heart beat faster and higher. This lends a certain lightness to the pursuit of even the biggest goals. True enthusiasm is a motivation welling up from the deepest layers of our being, allowing us to conquer the world like a fresh spring wind. Genuine enthusiasm trumps diligence and talent, and it provides a level of energy so that even unpleasant tasks are fulfilled with ease. What you do with enthusiasm and passion, you will do well, and what you do well will in most cases bring success of whatever nature. You play your own game, according to your own rules. You are the creator of your reality. That's the genuine expression of strong heart energy.

Those who go about life with passion also tend to be happier since by identifying with their actions they are able to see a higher meaning in what they do. This is both visible and palpable: such people are on fire; they glow, they shine, they sparkle. When they laugh, it's from the bottom of their very big heart. That's why they have space for others in their hearts. They have charisma and are like magnets. They are able to cast a spell over those around them and win their hearts – hearts that veritably fly towards them. They are a source of inspiration, especially for those in whom the life principle of the heart is only poorly developed.

Without the spark of inspiration and the fire of enthusiasm, life feels like a long winter. The lightness of summer is missing, as is its openness, its sensuality, its excitement. Everything is grey; the soul is starving, devoid of fun, listless, meaningless. The emperor is not at home; the spirit is on leave. For this reason, we may be looking to the outside world for a substitute, for someone to give our heart to. Weak heart energy is particularly prone to attach its heart to something or someone so that it can bring into the house the fire it's incapable of lighting itself. Such people need role models and heroes; they need a source of inspiration and an emperor to tell them which way to go. Unfortunately, this does not always work out well. Because you're listening not to your own heart but to that of others. Because you follow the light of others so that you can bask in their reflected glory. Once you've given away your heart, you've relinquished conscious control of your own life. It's easy to be manipulated and influenced. You're no longer a creator but a follower. You're no longer the ruler of your own empire, but rather an official handling and processing the orders of others. This weakens your identity, and you lose your inner fire.

Without the inner fire as fuel for the soul, everyday life has to be upheld by willpower and discipline instead. This requires much energy; as a result, the pursuit of your activities is half-hearted and faltering so that what you get back is less than what you invest. You do what you need to do, but you're not enjoying what you're doing. You get tired and feel empty quickly; you burn out without ever having burned properly. Since your inspiration is lying dormant, it's also difficult to find new paths or solutions. You're groping in the dark. What's missing is the light of the heart. And the right questions: What do I enjoy? What do I find inspiring?

These are precisely the qualities that characterise a well-developed life principle of the heart meridian: that life represents a game with a high entertainment value; that it's possible to create our own reality if only we passionately follow our heart. If you constantly follow others, you'll have to reclaim your fire – ideally, through activities that have no higher purpose than serving the lightness of being. Once the spark has been reignited, the rest of the body can be set on fire, too.

Love and the Universe

According to TCM, the *shen* has two faces: it can manifest in the form of individual consciousness, the realm of self-perception. However, individual consciousness represents only a limited form of expressing universal consciousness, which in TCM is referred to as *yuan shen*. The *yuan shen* is the ocean. The *shen* is the wave. The wave has individuality; it forms a separate unit. And yet it is a small part of a larger entity and couldn't even exist without it. The wave is a part of a supraordinate unit, being nourished and carried by it. A well-developed heart meridian results in a great and open heart, along with great and open awareness that doesn't end at the tip of one's nose. While the heart meridian experiences itself as a wave, it has a notion that it is part of an ocean. It enjoys pursuing this notion as it feels a subtle, yet extremely pleasant longing to connect with something bigger. It knows that precisely such a connectedness is required to feel truly carried and nourished by life, and to progress to deeper levels of contentment and finding meaning. The heart meridian needs an ocean in order to fully evolve.

A poorly developed life principle of the heart meridian engages only half-heartedly in the search for this ocean, often giving up once it has entered into a relationship where it's easy to experience feelings of attachment and being a unit, especially in the beginning. When in love or at the moment of orgasm, even the most blinkered *shen* is able to experience the meaning of time and space expanding, of two waves merging in an ocean. You merge to become one heart and one soul. That is the beginning. If you manage to stabilise this feeling and sustain it to become a settled relationship, it is entirely possible to create a supraordinate unit with another human, a supportive and caring relationship providing a sense of purpose. This is a state we generally refer to as love, and it is also love that opens our heart, letting it become expansive, so that there is space for more than just 'little me'. And because there is so much more out there, it's genuinely worthwhile not to listen to 'little me' and keep searching for the ocean.

The problem is that a heart meridian that's not fully developed may well open the door to let the other person in but then quickly close it again. It may even lock the door to preserve the feeling of oneness and connectedness till death do us part. We take our partner into our heart. We keep them locked in, which is quite a risky endeavour. When we are clinging to someone or something with all our heart, it's not love but desire. We hang on so tightly that the heart feels constricted. Or we can even lose our heart when the ocean we are so committed to begins to shift direction, and we become utterly lost in its vastness. Suddenly, the curtain rises to the big drama of lovesickness and heartache. A poorly developed life principle of the heart meridian may express itself in exaggerated jealousy and manic possessiveness, accompanied by separation anxiety and mistrust, control mechanisms, doubt and hypersensitivity. Without ocean, no water, and without water, no wave: I can't live without you, my sunshine, my heart, my everything. It feels like being annihilated by lovesickness. The reaction is fear, panic, rage, hatred, pain. The heart is broken and poisoned. These are not just phrases. Broken heart syndrome does actually exist.

Broken heart syndrome is a sudden-onset disorder of the heart muscle triggered by great emotional stress, such as separation, death, trauma or life-threatening situations. The symptoms are similar to a heart attack with concomitant cardiac insufficiency. The difference is that broken heart syndrome will generally heal by itself within a few weeks, depending on the intensity of the causative trigger. A well-developed heart meridian is the best immunity because it not only sees in another person the wave, but also recognises the ocean. It forms a unit with the wave and loves it very much in the knowledge that ultimately every wave will break. There can only be true peace in the heart when the heart meridian rises above the limitations of space and time, when the *shen* is carried by the *yuan shen*.

A big heart is characterised by its wise and often spiritual disposition, which is supported by its partner meridian, the small intestine. A heart like this is so big that it feels inherently connected with life; it feels carried by life. It is so big that it always has something to give. It is in love with all aspects of existence, with joy and suffering alike. It is calm and forbearing, and it loves for love's sake. It is both a wave and an ocean: the completion of the development of the heart meridian.

Signs of an Imbalanced and Balanced Heart Meridian

Signs of an Imbalanced Heart Meridian

- Little capacity for enthusiasm, little *joie de vivre*, little joyfulness
- Difficulty expressing oneself, mumbled or unclear speech
- A closed heart, emotionally reserved, difficulty opening up
- But also: hypersensitive, extremely emotional, very touchy
- Jealous, anxious, possessive in regard to relationships
- Hyperactive, unfocussed, nervous, forgetful, confused
- Easily breaking into a sweat, tendency to insomnia

Signs of a Balanced Heart Meridian

- Clear, focussed, concentrated, excellent comprehension
- A source of inspiration for self and others; enthusiastic, committed
- Consider themselves as creators of their own life; playing one's own game
- Emotionally independent and stable; outgoing and sociable, warm and sincere
- Charismatic, magnetic personality, emperor
- Interested in a meaningful life and a greater understanding of self and the world

How to Strengthen the Life Principle of the Heart Meridian

The Pleasure of Play

The inventors of the game 'Word Trio' had a deep understanding of the heart meridian. This game supports everything that makes the heart beat faster: great intellectual grasp, multi-level communication, astute mental and social activities, connectedness, team spirit. Playing this game will quickly reveal how free and liberated our heart energy really is. And it will support its cultivation. The heart enjoys fun and lightness. All the children of this world can't be wrong. Childhood is a time when the heart energy is very dominant, and nothing can get children more enthusiastic than playing. If this sounds perhaps a bit mundane and simplistic to you, just start playing a bit more. A few factors should be considered, though: no digital games, no gambling, and chess is a bit beside the point, too. Any game that's interactive and brings people together in a jolly way is a good start. Don't be tense. Let yourself be entertained.

Taking a Postprandial Nap

The emperor needs his rest in order to compose himself. A postprandial nap works wonders for strengthening the heart energy. According to the organ clock, noon is the time of the heart meridian, an excellent time for providing some rest for the heart but also for strengthening it. A little break improves concentration and memory, both aspects of the heart meridian. In the long term, a daily ration of sleep at noon can lower the risk of heart disease by 30%. In particular, those prone to a somewhat sensitive heart should make use of any opportunity to gather the *shen*'s dissolute energy. Please note: do not sleep for more than half an hour, or the body will enter the slow-wave sleep phase. A couch or comfortable chair is better than lying down in bed. The room should not be too dark so that it's easier to wake up again. Not possible during your working hours? Hands on the desk, head on the hands, and you're ready for bit of napping. That's not possible either? There's no excuse at the weekend! Sleep well.

The Pathway of the Heart Meridian

The heart meridian arises in a depression in the centre of the armpit, the location of Heart 1. From here, the meridian courses in an almost straight line in a groove along the inner triceps (triceps brachii) to reach Heart 3. With the elbow bent, Heart 3 can be found at the inner end of the elbow crease. The heart meridian continues by traversing the medial (ulnar) muscles of the forearm in a slight curve. The closer the heart meridian gets to the wrist, the closer it gets to the ulna, travelling in a groove between the ulna and the tendon of the ulnar-side hand flexor (flexor carpi ulnaris), which runs towards the pisiform bone. Heart 7 is on the wrist crease, slightly below the pisiform bone.

The heart meridian traverses the palm in the direction of the little finger, following a groove between the fourth and fifth metacarpal bones. Heart 8 can be found next to the fifth metacarpal bone, where the little finger comes to rest when the fist is clenched. The meridian continues along the fifth metacarpal bone to course along the inside of the little finger to Heart 9, located on the thumb-side corner of the nail of the little finger.

Key Areas of the Heart Meridian

Axilla

The heart meridian begins in a depression in the centre of the axilla at Heart 1, *ji quan* or 'Summit Spring'. The armpits are a good indicator of the status of the heart energy: Is the heart calm and stable? Is it nervous and insecure? The heart meridian belongs to the fire element, which tends to express any imbalances through heat symptoms. We begin to sweat, sometimes very intensely. The heart is agitated. The armpits are a very intimate area of the body, just as the heart is a very intimate organ. It can be embarrassing when huge, damp patches begin to form around Heart 1. And it is often also experienced as uncomfortable to open the armpits as this is a state in which the heart meridian is extremely vulnerable. It's for a reason that the command for exposing or disarming someone is 'Hands up!' Generally, bringing our hands up and folding them comfortably behind our head is a posture we only assume when we feel safe and relaxed. Ostentatiously crossing the arms behind the head can also be seen as a demonstration of power: 'Look at me, my heart is so strong that I don't need to hide it. I am the "Summit Spring"!' Conversely, we close and protect our heart by pressing our arms across our chest: no access to Heart 1, no access to the origin of the heart meridian. We close the spring of the heart.

Hands

Besides the face, eyes and tongue, the hands are a further important key area of the heart. Like the heart, the hands can be hard or soft, lively or tired. We can reach out to someone with an open hand or we can hit them in the face with a fist. By opening and closing our hands, we also open and close our heart. A strong heart meridian provides the hands with much energy so that they are warm and soft. Without this energy the hands remain cold. A weak heart can manifest in a restless and nervous demeanour, expressed in shaky or sweaty hands. The most important point for calming the heart can be found on the wrist crease. Heart 7, *shen men* or 'Spirit Gate', allows us to directly address our *shen*, our awareness. *Shen men* is an excellent point for calming the *shen* when there is anxiety and stress. The heart meridian terminates at the little finger, the most sensitive of all the fingers. This, too, mirrors the subtle heart energy. Among the Japanese Yakuza it was an old custom to cut off a part of the little finger and offer it to one's superior: offering a part of the heart as a symbolic admission of guilt.

The Heart Meridian: Key Points

- Associated element: Fire element
- Quality: Yin
- Time on the organ clock: 11am–1pm
- Animal quality: Horse
- Partner meridian: Small intestine meridian
- Twinned meridian: Kidney meridian
- Opposite meridian: Gallbladder meridian

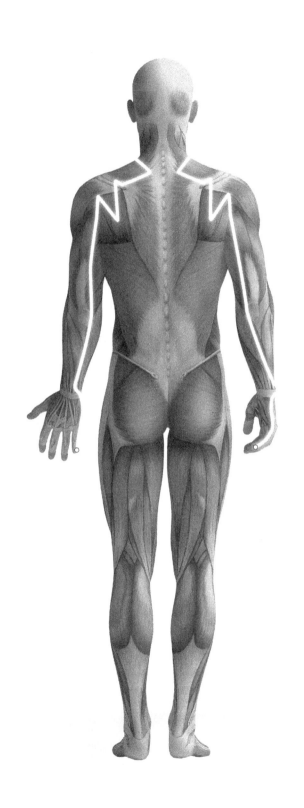

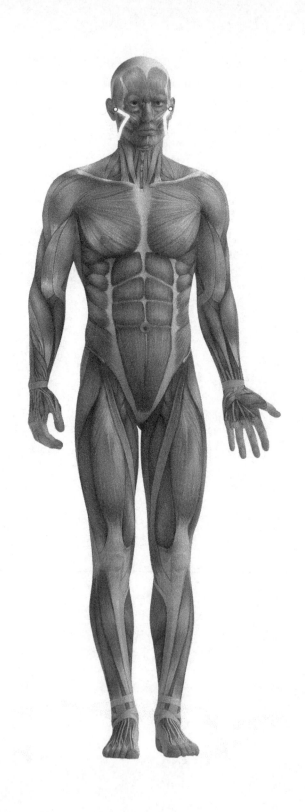

Chapter 9

The Small Intestine Meridian

Discerning Clarity

Questions for the Small Intestine Meridian

- Do I have access to spirituality?
- Do I feel embedded in something bigger?
- Do I feel supported and carried by something bigger?
- Am I able to feel a deep connectedness with other people or with life?
- Do I grasp things easily?
- Can I think and learn quickly? Can I get quickly to the point?
- Do I easily feel mentally overwhelmed?
- Am I sometimes confused, losing my orientation in life?
- Am I able to discern between the important and the unimportant?
- Do I tend to distinguish between thoughts and feelings?
- Do I sometimes feel isolated and not understood?
- Am I often over-critical? Can I be rash in categorising?

The Life Principle of the Small Intestine Meridian

In TCM, the task of the small intestine is to separate the clear from the turbid. The clear is absorbed from ingested food and integrated into the body. The turbid is passed on further for elimination. In a simplified way, this corresponds to the digestive processes on a physical level. However, the small intestine meridian is destined for better things. It is responsible for separating the clear from the turbid on all levels. The task of separating a clouded way of seeing from pure perception makes the small intestine the most spiritual of all meridians. It separates illusion from insight so that the true nature of being can be recognised and comprehended.

The life principle of the small intestine meridian opens us up to the higher dimensions and deeper meaning of life. Without the small intestine meridian, we lack the connection to the mystical, to an invisible 'more', to a supraordinate, all-permeating entity. The small intestine meridian allows us to look beyond the tips of our noses and experience ourselves as part of a greater whole, resulting in a feeling of deep connectedness with others and with life. It's about growth and yet more growth, until growth goes beyond the self. When this aspect is missing in our lives, an inner emptiness will gnaw away at our souls despite material abundance, despite freedom and self-actualisation, despite health and contentment. We may have reached the zenith of our life, but how do we continue from there? What can life still have in store for us? The life principle of the small intestine provides the answers.

The small intestine's function of separating is also of crucial importance in everyday life. As the partner meridian of the heart, the small intestine is also concerned with clarity. While the clarity of the heart is soft and loving, that of the small intestine is razor-sharp and precise. It stands for presence of mind, the capacity for quick comprehension and straight judgement. If the life principle of the small intestine is well developed, it is able to separate what is important for it and what isn't, without any hesitation. The result is great efficiency in daily life: you're able to recognise, set and stick with priorities. You don't get bogged down, you don't get scattered. You get straight to the point without pussyfooting about, sometimes perhaps a little bit too directly and harshly where interpersonal relations are concerned since an imbalanced small intestine meridian can be expressed in an underlying know-it-all manner and hypercritical thinking. In that case, thoughts are likely to be divisive rather than connecting. We run the risk of tunnel vision because reflection isn't considered. As the act of separating becomes all-consuming, we may even become deluded so that we can only see one truth: our own.

This kind of separation can potentially lead to feelings of insecurity since you constantly isolate yourself and don't properly belong anywhere. You turn into a habitual loner who feels misunderstood and unloved. In addition, a malfunctioning small intestine tends to separate thoughts from feelings and feelings from thoughts. You and your life become fragmented, until there's a heap of separate areas unconnected with each other. You can't see the forest for the trees.

In contrast, a small intestine with a well-developed life principle not only sees the forest but sees the soil in which it is rooted; it sees the sky providing it with water, the animals living therein. This leads to deep contentment because you're carried by the strong feeling that you are more than just this forest, more than just the interface of one awareness and one body. Such people have no need to push the fulfilment of their personal requirements or their ego to the foreground all the time. They know they can be effective in a quiet way and are happy to go to the end of the queue. They find fulfilment by subordinating their actions and their aspirations to a greater whole. They have the capacity to transcend themselves.

The life principle of the small intestine meridian is an extremely important building block of life. Only the integration of a spiritual dimension can lead us to genuine contentment and health. Without a small intestine meridian, we would be merely scratching the surface of our existence.

The Small Intestine Meridian and the Body

The Strength Within

Partially digested food remains for many hours in the small intestine, which can be up to six metres long. It absorbs about 90% of nutrients. According to TCM, it's the task of the small intestine to extract the so-called precious essences and to supply them to our body. The clear is absorbed. The turbid is passed on. A healthy separating function results in vitality, physical robustness and a strong immune system. Problems arise when the small intestine lacks the clarity required for separating so that it separates too much or too little. This results in a weakness regarding absorption and assimilation. In other words, the small intestine finds it hard to filter and integrate from the ingested food what the body needs. It can easily be overwhelmed by this task, and this will impair digestion, resulting in bloating, sensations of fullness and diarrhoea. In severe cases, this can lead to a state of malabsorption and deficiency symptoms. The body becomes weakened. It gains too little energy and has to draw on its resources.

It's the same on a psychological level. From the stream of information and emotions impacting on it, a weak small intestine meridian is incapable of filtering out what is genuinely relevant and useful. What is unimportant is deemed important, and vice versa. Affected people may therefore have problems with mental processing and accordingly may find it difficult to bring order and structure to their thinking patterns. The result is a bloated head that feels full, a kind of mental diarrhoea, or, put differently, confusion, nervousness, difficulties concentrating or forgetfulness. Furthermore, if the filter provided by the small intestine fails, we are helplessly exposed to the relentless bombardment of the modern information society. We are susceptible to being hopelessly sucked into the vortex of social media. Every day, we consume a plethora of tiny information titbits that pass through our bodies without any true nutritional value. At the same time, we're unable to read an entire book because we can't maintain our focus for more than a few minutes. We distract ourselves at every possible opportunity with every possible app. We welcome digital games at the level of a child. Anything more than that and our limp small intestine simply can't cope.

A further imbalance of the small intestine meridian expresses itself in an exaggerated separating function. In such cases, the small intestine is hypersensitive and separates too vehemently, quickly rejecting things such as certain foods or certain ingredients – for example, dairy, gluten or fructose. It has no use for these substances and, being unable to absorb or process them, it responds with allergies and heat when exposed to them. This is often the starting point for many inflammatory bowel diseases (IBD). Most of these disorders are congenital but become worse when the body is stressed so that the small intestine gets overwhelmed on a mental level with absorption and assimilation, which leaves even less energy to be invested in the gastrointestinal tract. A small vicious circle: a weakness in the small intestine leads to a weakness in the capacity for psychological processing, leads to becoming stressed more quickly, leads to further irritation of the small intestine, leads to further weakness. What helps is calmness and clarity in matters of lifestyle and diet. A clear separation of what is good for you and what isn't.

A well-functioning life principle of the small intestine meridian provides strength and equanimity for both digestion and the mental realm. This is a small intestine that knows precisely what to pick from what's on offer in order to benefit from it. Anything burdensome isn't allowed to enter in the first place. It can therefore also be seen as a gatekeeper who rejects what doesn't serve. It can afford to do that as it is able to make much out of little. People with a strong small intestine energy are extremely good at processing food and they are extremely sharp thinkers. They find it easy to grasp and process the essence of complex matters. They know what has to be taken in and passed on further. This provides clarity: in the gut, in the head, in life.

SYMPTOMS ASSOCIATED WITH THE SMALL INTESTINE MERIDIAN

Digestive disorders, chronic inflammatory bowel diseases (Crohn's disease, ulcerative colitis...), malabsorption, food allergies and intolerances (coeliac disease, lactose, fructose...), nutritional deficiencies, fatigue, poor immunity...

This Thing About the Pipes

In some people, the small intestine separates with too much vigour and rigidity. In others, it does so too little and too rashly as it is unsure what is clear and what is turbid and prefers to let everything in, taking everything on. The body gets flooded by such undifferentiated absorption, and the gastrointestinal tract becomes overwhelmed. The small intestine swallows it all but doesn't utilise it. A hopelessly swamped compost heap builds up inside the belly. Congestion, fermentation and putrefaction set in. In TCM, we talk about a toxic overload: turbid food waste instead of clear nutritional essence. This waste is responsible for the congestion of important pathways.

Imagine the following scenario: a central heating system in which heavily contaminated sludge circulates instead of water. It is only a matter of time until the pipes become clogged up. The central nervous system, including the brain, corresponds to the pipes. The small intestine is responsible for the purity of the fluids. When the small intestine energy is weakened and doesn't sufficiently separate the clear from the turbid, there will be a build-up of metabolic waste resulting from the poor processing. Over the years and decades, a ticking timebomb builds up. Whether it's schizophrenia or mania, Parkinson's or Alzheimer's disease, according to TCM, it's all a problem of blocked, corroded or poisoned pathways. It all originates in the small intestine. But once the pathways are contaminated to such an extent, it's generally too late. Prevention is thus the best alternative, which is also a function of the small intestine's life principle: to keep the turbid outside the door. The clarity of a balanced small intestine meridian helps to lead life with awareness as it knows that every effect has a cause. It has an excellent ability for sound judgement and reasoning.

A robust small intestine energy results in a clear and focussed lifestyle that is based on insight and awareness rather than on rigidly following certain rules or guidelines. Such people appreciate health and vitality, and consistently avoid detrimental influences. Discipline and persistency regarding diet, exercise and mental focus come easily and without any trouble. They part with unnecessary ballast that prevents the pursuit of long-term goals.

A disordered small intestine meridian, on the other hand, will act completely differently because it doesn't know where to draw the line: chaos reigns, in the gut, in the head, in the fridge, in the home. The environment mirrors the gut: mess everywhere – we're reminded of the obsessively amassing and accumulating hoarder.

Hoarders can't let go of anything, and piles of rubbish gradually form in all the different areas of their lives. Often they don't even notice what's going on. It's not just material things that are hoarded, but also tasks or social commitments that build up and create a logjam. The conscious capacity to act diminishes more and more, crushed by tons of redundant clutter. Life's pathways are clogged up, and the ability for sound judgement and evaluation no longer exists. Any clarity in the head is paralysed by the polluted abdominal brain in the form of the small intestine. Our consciousness is clouded. Unobscured perspectives have become impossible.

In TCM, there is an image that sees the small intestine as the yellow springs in the interior of the earth. Yellow is the colour of the earth element, the element of the centre. And these springs are in the earth's interior, in the centre of the centre, so to speak. In the event of big problems, people would turn to these springs as they are the abode of the ancestors with all their knowledge and wisdom. Symbolically speaking, this means that when dealing with important questions, don't just listen to your head but also to your gut. The belly is where the small intestine takes up a central location. It's for a reason that the small intestine is also referred to as the 'abdominal brain'. Even the visual similarity with the brain is obvious. When the life principle of the small intestine is well developed, the gut will know better than the head what is good for you and what isn't. And the belly will also let you know this, by way of good intuition and a good feeling towards yourself. We're more likely to stay away from doing silly things that could harm us. We instinctively keep our pathways clean. This is the foundation for a conscious lifestyle and long-term health, which, as is well known, begins in the gut.

SYMPTOMS ASSOCIATED WITH THE SMALL INTESTINE MERIDIAN

Emotional and/or mental restlessness, confusion, developmental disorders, mental illness, split personality disorder, hoarding syndrome, impaired speech, neurodegenerative disorders such as Alzheimer's or Parkinson's disease...

The Small Intestine Meridian and the Psyche

Clear, Not So Clear, Higgledy-Piggledy

It is part of the life principle of the small intestine to separate the clear from the turbid. The result is clarity. Imagine a glass full of mud. Because of the cloudiness, hardly anything can be recognised. In and of itself, the water would be clear were it not so contaminated. The small intestine separates the turbid parts from the clear water; it is the ultimate filter for our perception, thought processes and analyses. Suddenly, you can see clearly and the penny drops, because consciousness, by its nature, would be clear, were it not constantly muddied by the myriad influences that everyday life brings in its wake. Here, too, the small intestine can create order.

However, when the small intestine is imbalanced, it lacks this trait. Our mind is unable to discern between important and unimportant stimuli and input. It finds it difficult to differentiate one thought from another, one emotion from another. In addition, thoughts are mistaken for emotions and emotions for thoughts. Reality and imagination may be mixed up as well. A jumble arises in the head, and confusion and bewilderment spread. This has far-reaching consequences: the chaotic mess muddles our consciousness. In TCM, many cognitive abilities are directly associated with the small intestine meridian. An imbalance in the meridian can manifest as difficulties with reading, writing, listening, learning or understanding. Many forms of delayed childhood development or mental illness have their roots in our abdominal brain, the small intestine. Less pronounced forms show up as disorientation, disorganisation or a latent stupor. You're not quite with it. You don't even know where you actually are or what's happening with your thoughts and your perception. You find it hard to process and understand what's going on around you.

You appear a little bit like a two-legged cow surprised by life. Everyday life turns into an obstacle course; even small tasks can turn into a huge challenge. You feel easily overwhelmed, mentally exhausted. Your focus goes down the drain, it's hard to concentrate and productivity suffers. Five minutes of attention is all you can muster. Then you need some distraction: a quick glance at your phone or checking your emails for the umpteenth time, in the hope a new one may have appeared, promising a worthwhile surprise. Self-management, as well as managing time and priorities, is particularly fraught with difficulties. You find it challenging to keep your life in order and well organised. You've ended up in a jungle and are no longer on top of things.

A robust small intestine meridian would act completely differently. Its mind plays on the level of a samurai. It sees precisely what is going on, unadulterated, crystal clear and fast. Every situation or experience is consciously and comprehensively processed rather than habitually evaluated based on emotions or engrained behavioural patterns. Based on a well-developed perceptiveness, the small intestine is able to assess what is important and right. It can thus process the information gained and reach an appropriate conclusion: the prerequisite for clear judgement and clear decisions. This, in turn, leads to clear actions. A straight and plain talk. Words are followed by consistent endeavours – in other words, a high congruence between the internal and external world: you walk your talk, straight forward, unswervingly. The small intestine meridian is also the meridian of perseverance. No other meridian endows us with such strong stamina and such clear orientation towards our goal. It is the marathon meridian.

The process of separating can, of course, be carried to extremes so that the thinking becomes compartmentalised, and the world is seen in black and white only. There are no nuances, no grey zones, no 'as well as', only pigeonholes unconnected with each other. And, most importantly, no mingling of feelings and thoughts. The energy gets stuck in the head; emotions are not allowed. Such people find it hard to be socially integrated or enter into meaningful relationships as they are not very willing to compromise because they subject everything to reason. To others, they appear cold, hard and dismissive. An overzealous small intestine represents a direct path towards dissatisfaction. Life is wrecked by overthinking. It gets dissected, torn apart. It lacks softness, *joie de vivre*, silliness.

Yet it's precisely the life principle of the small intestine meridian that ensures deep mental peace and inner calm. Strong small intestine energy is able to alight from the merry-go-round of thinking; it won't let itself be distracted or influenced by fears rooted in the past and worries about the future. The path of clarity will always also lead to the self. And in the next step beyond the self.

Spirituality and Transcendence

Spirituality is a basic human need. There is no society or people that has not spawned some form of belief system or religion. Spirituality is based on the subliminal feeling that there could be more to life and this planet, something that cannot quite be grasped or fathomed. Even people who claim that spirituality means nothing to them know this feeling. Every now and again, they feel a longing in their soul, perhaps in nature, perhaps in stillness, sometimes after particularly intense events. They feel this every time their boundaries begin to loosen and widen. Spirituality can be seen as the desire to connect with something bigger than oneself. The life principle of the small intestine ensures that you connect with what is right for you.

The small intestine separates; that is its function. But its function is also to divest itself of the illusion of separation, which in itself is the expression of a disordered small intestine meridian. If it separates too vehemently, then you become separated from life, from other people, from the exchange with others, from connectedness. The result is that you become too focussed on your own self, on your ego, as it is referred to in many spiritual traditions, which recognise it as the root of all evil. Those who only identify with themselves, only see themselves, are ultimately alone. They are the sun in the centre of their very own solar system and in love with their very own light while ignoring the shadows. The lynchpin of their world view is their own ideas and convictions, which are, of course, sacrosanct and to which they cling at all costs. The preferred strategy of an imbalanced small intestine is to come up with a construct that allows for constant self-validation as there is nothing else it could use to define itself. Anything that may threaten this construct is considered a danger and fought against. The bigger the ego, the bigger the fear of losing it. This, however, will inevitably happen, at the latest at the time of death. Buddhism sees the exaggerated clinging to the idea of a fixed self as the root of all suffering. The cure is awareness and insight. And who takes care of these? The small intestine!

A small intestine meridian with a well-developed life principle endows us with the ability to recognise that we are all more or less in the same boat. All beings want to be happy, all beings want to grow. To this end, everybody is looking for their individual path. Some paths may appear a bit bizarre; others may never lead to the goal. The small intestine doesn't see the paths. Rather, it sees the human being walking these paths; it sees what moves a person, what they truly seek, what they truly want, be it a fighter pilot or a pool attendant. The clearer the small intestine meridian, the clearer the insight, sometimes to the point of realising that our deep desire for contentment connects us all, that we are not on our own with this longing, that we all desire safety and love. The clearer the small intestine, the stronger the connectedness, not only with other people but also with nature as it is an illusion to experience ourselves separate from either.

We need clean air for breathing, we need clean water for drinking, we need a climate in which we can grow crops; we need a healthy environment for survival, and we are much more a part of our environment than we tend to believe. The small intestine recognises this. It considers itself a part of the enormous ecosystem of planet earth, an intrinsic part of nature, which it sees as neither foe nor a self-service shop. This results in mindful and responsible behaviour so characteristic of people with a strong small intestine energy. They have the capacity to care. They can think way beyond the end of their nose, and not only that, they also feel and understand things on a very deep level of their consciousness. They transcend the narrow boundaries of their self-centredness. They find meaning beyond their individual development. This represents a fundamental spiritual attitude.

Based on such a spiritual attitude, a small intestine with a well-developed life principle is able to divest itself of any categorising, judgemental or stereotyping behaviour. It is able to liberate itself and to put the fulfilment of personal needs and the maximisation of any benefits on the back burner. It is able to strive for a deep commitment to higher goals that are beyond the self. It is able to advocate altruistically for the benefit of the community and social justice because it feels connected to the collective, holistic development of the world. This connectedness contributes to the small intestine being able to perceive and experience its existence as meaningful.

Lacking these experiences represents a weakness of the small intestine meridian. A person will have a vague feeling of missing something, even if all personal and material needs are largely satisfied. This missing something can gnaw away at someone's happiness since there is no meaning in life and the soul is starving. The good news: there is no need to look for meaning outside of oneself. It can be found right inside of us. And the icing on the cake: to feel connected not only to other people, to humanity, to nature and all sentient beings but to something that no one can really name, with a force that serves as a carrier for all visible and invisible manifestations. Religions use the term 'deity' in this context. In TCM, it is referred to as the *dao*. At this point, it may be helpful to simply speak of magic. Anyone who has ever gazed at the starlit sky with clear small intestine energy will have had a glimpse of this.

Signs of an Imbalanced and Balanced Small Intestine Meridian

Signs of an Imbalanced Small Intestine Meridian

- Frequent feelings of being isolated, alone and disconnected
- Getting confused easily, quick to lose a sense of orientation
- Often feeling dull and dazed in the head
- Difficulties with separating and connecting thoughts and feelings
- Unable to differentiate and set priorities
- Often over-critical, being a know-all, likes to pigeonhole
- Tendency to food allergies and intolerances
- Egocentric attitudes based on feelings of insecurity

Signs of a Balanced Small Intestine Meridian

- Able to look beyond the self and one's own world view
- Able to connect with a deeper meaning and wider-reaching tasks
- Feels embedded in and carried by life, able to access spirituality
- Able to act and be active in a social and sustainable manner
- Able to think quickly, sharply and clearly, able to get to the point and set priorities
- Able to learn well, grasp and integrate new things

How to Strengthen the Life Principle of the Small Intestine Meridian

Journaling

Journaling refers to the writing down of thoughts, feelings and events – it is a kind of diary. The difference is that journaling follows a set, repetitive routine. This helps the mind to find order and structure. At the same time, journaling provides clarity, which is something the small intestine really likes. It is important to write by hand. Compared with typing on a keyboard, writing by hand stimulates a significantly larger number of areas in the brain, which in turn leads to a much stronger cross-linking of information. We understand much better what we have written by hand. In addition, it is really helpful to perform the ritual of journaling always at the same time – the morning and evening are best. Three minutes is sufficient. Define three questions that you aim to pursue over a period of time, for example: What did I enjoy today? What did I get annoyed about today? What am I grateful for? You can choose random themes. What's important is the routine. There are a wide range of journaling diaries available covering different areas of life, with specified questions and a specified format. They provide a good way of getting started. The small intestine will certainly like this exercise.

Get Connected

Every day, look for a person with whom to do this exercise. It doesn't have to be someone you know. It can be any person at all, someone you meet during the course of the day, perhaps at work or in the street. What's important: choose the person randomly and not according to your preferences or aversions. A little helpful trick: set a time, for example, 8.15am. At exactly that time, you do the exercise with the person standing next to you. Look at this person, not so much with your eyes but with your heart. Gather your focus in your chest area and try to get a real sense of that person. They are a human being, just like you. A human being who's trying to be happy, who wants to express their personality, who's striving for meaning and safety. This person does it their own way, just as you are doing it in yours. Ultimately, you both have the same desire, the same motivation; only your approach will be different, perhaps even completely different. But there is more that connects you than separates you. Try to feel this connectedness. Once every day.

The Pathway of the Small Intestine Meridian

The small intestine meridian begins at Small Intestine 1 on the lateral aspect of the little finger, at the corner of the nail. It courses along the outside border of the little finger, at the border of the palmar and dorsal aspects to Small Intestine 3, located at the end of the crease that forms in this area by making a fist. It continues along the side of the hand to Small Intestine 4, which can be found in a depression between the joint of the fifth metacarpal bone and the pisiform bone.

The meridian crosses the bony protrusion at the distal end of the ulna (styloid process), coursing closely along the upper edge of the ulna to Small Intestine 8, located in a depression on the back of the elbow, between the olecranon and the medial epicondyle of the humerus. It continues across the medial head of the triceps towards the shoulder and Small Intestine 9, a point one thumb-width above the axillary fold. From here, the meridian ascends perpendicularly to the lower border of the scapular spine, the location of Small Intestine 10. The small intestine meridian now runs towards the centre of the scapula, the location of Small Intestine 11. From there, it ascends almost perpendicularly in the direction of the shoulder and traverses the scapular spine, where Small Intestine 12 is located in a depression (fossa supraspinata) above the scapular spine. At the medial end of this fossa lies Small Intestine 13. From here, the small intestine meridian courses towards the seventh cervical vertebra. Small Intestine 15 lies two thumb-widths lateral to the spinous process of the seventh cervical vertebra.

The small intestine meridian now curves around the lower part of the neck towards the anterior and in doing so crosses the trapezius. It then ascends the lateral aspect of the neck and crosses the sternocleidomastoid to reach Small Intestine 17. This point is located behind the jaw angle, on the anterior border of the sternocleidomastoid, on a vertical line beneath the ear lobe. As it continues further, the small intestine meridian traverses the lower jawbone to course anteriorly on the lateral aspect of the face. Small Intestine 18 can be found below the cheekbone, on a line running perpendicularly from the lateral corner of the eye. From there, the meridian travels along the lower border of the cheekbone back to the ear where Small Intestine 19 is situated in a depression that can be palpated when the mouth is slightly open.

Key Areas of the Small Intestine Meridian

Lower Abdomen

The point Ren Mai 4, *guan yuan* or 'Origin Pass', is located on the lower abdomen, three thumb-widths below the navel. This area also represents the diagnostic zone of the kidney meridian on the abdomen. The fact that Ren Mai 4 is also the alarm point of the small intestine clearly demonstrates the close connection between it and the kidneys. Both the small intestine and the kidneys are strongly involved with the *yuan qi*. The small intestine produces *yuan qi* by extracting the pure essence from ingested food, and the kidneys store it. The area around Ren Mai 4 is a good indicator of whether the store is full or empty, and also of the body's actual energy reserves. When this area is empty, the resources are scarce, too: a red flag that the small intestine is not really able to fulfil its task, assimilating too little essence during the digestive process. Therefore, the kidneys don't receive anything they could store.

But it can also happen that a weakened life principle of the small intestine results in the gut being separated from the rest of the body, so that we live purely from the head, avoiding a connection with our feelings or our true centre. If this is the case, the lower abdomen will appear weak and empty because it doesn't get any attention or any energy. Conversely, it can happen that we find fullness at Ren Mai 4. However, this fullness is often an expression of deficiency: the small intestine doesn't separate well enough; it takes in everything without reflection so that the body becomes flooded, leading to stagnation. The kidneys get drowned in this flood, which disturbs their life principle. When the clarity of the small intestine is missing and the mind is clouded, it will be difficult to answer typical kidney questions such as 'Who am I?' and 'What do I want?' In either scenario, Ren Mai 4 is an excellent point to strengthen this area so important for the small intestine.

Shoulder Blade

The shoulder blade is the origin of the rotator cuff, a group of four muscles whose tendons form a cap that almost completely encloses the head of the humerus. Stabilising the shoulder joint is an important function of the rotator cuff. Although it has a wide range of motion, the shoulder is much less stable than the hip joint, as its bony fixation is much weaker. The free movement of the shoulder joint reflects the flexibility of the heart and mind. After all, hand on heart, we express ourselves by using our arms and hands, we talk with our hands, we take things to heart; with our arms and hands, we hug, shape and form. This corresponds to the quality of the fire element, which includes the small intestine. Its task with regard to the shoulder joint is to be clear about what is the right time and the right place to open up or to close.

Too much openness is associated with a weakness of the separating function of the small intestine. Without hesitation or reflection, we open up to everything and anything, we let everything get close to us, we don't really know how to defend ourselves. This often goes hand in hand with a hyperflexible shoulder joint. Conversely, when there is tightness and tension in the rotator cuff, the shoulder joint can be closed with only a limited range of motion, clearly manifesting in the form of shoulder pain. This is typical of a small intestine whose separating function is overwhelmed. It separates too much and closes itself off from too many things.

In the centre of the shoulder blade we find the point Small Intestine 11, *tian zong* or 'Celestial Gathering'. Small Intestine 11 expresses whether we are able to align ourselves with heaven, whether we are able to truly commit to relationships. It expresses whether we are sufficiently open so that our awareness can expand beyond our ego to embrace what is beyond ourselves.

Side of the Hand

The small intestine meridian begins on the little finger and controls the side of the hand. The lateral aspect of our hands commands great strength for separating. Bricks and stones can be separated with one single karate chop. The side of the hand stands for focussed clarity. In this area, we also find the point Small Intestine 3, *hou xi* or 'Back Ravine', which is often needled for disorders along the entire small intestine meridian.

The Small Intestine Meridian: Key Points

- Associated element: Fire element
- Quality: Yang
- Time on the organ clock: 1pm–3pm
- Animal quality: Goat
- Partner meridian: Heart meridian
- Twinned meridian: Bladder meridian
- Opposite meridian: Liver meridian

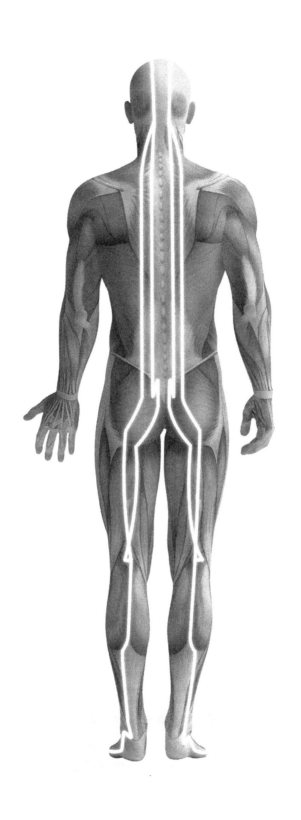

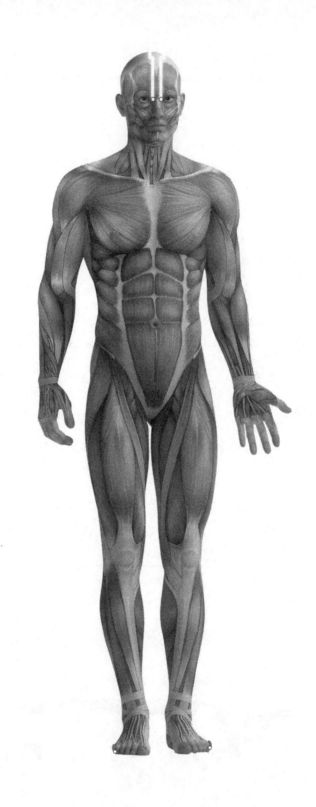

Chapter 10

The Bladder Meridian
Activity, Cleansing and Regeneration

Questions for the Bladder Meridian

- Am I able to get active easily? Do I quickly gain momentum?
- Am I able to relax during periods of rest?
- Am I able to compose and regenerate myself?
- Do I find it easy to alternate between tension and relaxation?
- Am I able to fight for something if required?
- Do I have strong nerves?
- Am I able to show calm and equanimity?
- Do I run away from things or bury my head in the sand?
- Am I able to allow and show emotions?
- Do I cope well with stress and emotional strain?
- Do I have a sensitive bladder?
- Am I prone to urinary tract infections?

The Life Principle of the Bladder Meridian

Without the bladder meridian, nothing would ever happen at all. We would be like a bicycle without wheels, like an engine without fuel, like a saddle without a horse. We wouldn't be getting anywhere; we would be rooted to the spot, stock-still and static, Sleeping Beauty in slow-wave sleep. The bladder meridian kisses us awake since the life principle of the bladder meridian stands for activity. It's the guy who pushes us, the instigator who makes sure that we move our backside off the couch and start doing, doing, doing... The bladder meridian is the key we need to start the motor called human being. It is the authority that ensures that high-octane fuel enriches our blood.

Of course, the key can also be used to switch the engine off again; that's important. Having a key for switching on the engine is all well and good, but overactive non-stop operation will wear down even the best engine constructed with the best materials. At some point, it'll simply pack in. So it's also part and parcel of the bladder meridian's life principle to take the foot off the accelerator at the right time and curb the speed when we have been on the go for too long or too intensely or too fast, unable to pace ourselves yet again. The bladder meridian not only ensures that we take necessary breaks, but also takes care that we truly relax and rejuvenate ourselves while we rest.

When the life principle of the bladder meridian is well developed, it allows us to switch effortlessly between activity and rest depending on what is required in a particular situation. We find it easy to gain momentum and equally easy to revert to relaxation. The bladder meridian pays attention that we stay in flux and don't get stuck in a particular operating mode, no matter what the circumstances demand of us. An imbalance in the life principle of the bladder meridian can result in us being unable to switch off during free periods or being unable to become active when this is required. We carry work stress over into our leisure time, and by the same token we bring inactivity to the workplace. Night turns into day, and day into night. This can lead to friction and turbulence. Over time, friction will always engender heat and waste products. In order to clear these up, we certainly need the bladder meridian.

In TCM, the bladder meridian is responsible for cleansing the body. Together with the kidneys, the bladder filters and eliminates any waste that burdens the body or no longer serves it. As always, TCM doesn't differentiate between matter and energy: too much uric acid in the blood is as dangerous as an excess of toxic emotions. Emotions become toxic when they exceed our capacity to consciously process them, with the result that they have the potential to poison us. In this context, the bladder serves as the authority for collecting and eliminating. It is the overflow basin for excess emotional strain: it protects us from running hot by safeguarding continuous filtering and elimination processes. It keeps us and our emotions in flux.

The bladder meridian shares a further aspect of its tasks with the kidney meridian. The bladder and the kidneys are both associated with the water element. It is the element of willpower, however, that is expressed differently by the bladder and kidneys. The kidney meridian stands for willpower that arises deep within our core and is activated by inner images and motives. In comparison, the willpower of the bladder meridian is relatively superficial. It acts for its own sake. It is determined to get its own way, regardless of whether that makes sense or not. Like a rider without pity or mercy, it can spur our body to the point of exhaustion and beyond. This kind of will stands for fight and confrontation. If the life principle of the bladder meridian is well developed, we can tap into its resources during big challenges or times of crises. But if the bladder meridian is weak, we react to even the slightest stress with flight and resignation.

The life principle of the bladder meridian energises us. If we have too little energy, we never gain momentum properly, while too much energy will lead us into burnout. Recognising and maintaining the right balance between the two is the hallmark of a healthy bladder meridian.

The Bladder Meridian and the Body

The Yin and Yang of the Nervous System

The pathway of the bladder meridian follows the most important sections of the central nervous system. It has its greatest influence on the head and spine, on the brain and spinal cord. The bladder meridian represents the autonomic nervous system with its two opposing aspects, thus beautifully mirroring the principles of yin and yang. The sympathetic nervous system starts up the body and brings it up to speed. It stands for the aspect of the bladder meridian that activates us and prepares us to act. It governs the yang. The parasympathetic nervous system returns the body to a state of relaxation so that we can rest and recharge our batteries. When we are tired or exhausted, it sends signals to the body that it needs to take a break, especially through sleep and the recovery that occurs during sleep. The parasympathetic division is justifiably referred to as the 'Lord of the Night'. It governs the yin. If the life principle of the bladder meridian is well developed, we can smoothly and effortlessly switch between different states, depending on what is required. But if the life principle of the bladder meridian is affected by an imbalance, it often happens that we tend to dwell too much in one state – with far-reaching consequences.

The sympathetic nervous system prepares our body for physical and mental activities. Once activated, the heart beats more strongly and faster, the airways dilate, stored energy is released, muscular strength increases and blood pressure rises in order to supply the body with more blood. At the same time, those physiological processes that do not benefit the activated state are reduced – for example, digestion and the desire to void the bladder. The actual purpose of this function is to facilitate flight or quick defence in case of danger. This mechanism is a remnant of primeval times when we were still confronted by genuine, tangible danger that required a physical response.

The problem is that times have changed but this automatic response has remained. When stress knocks on our door, the sympathetic nervous system throws itself against it and revs up the machine called human. A cocktail of hormones is released – adrenalin, noradrenalin, cortisol – and the nervous system works flat out. That's all fine as long as we're able to scale back the over-activation when the danger is over. If you were running away from a sabre-toothed tiger in the year dot, the stress was eliminated through the intense physical exertion. However, in our modern way of living, this metabolic mechanism is utilised too rarely and not to a sufficient degree. The stress remains in the body until it makes us sick. The fact that the bladder meridian is the only one to have so-called back-*shu* points (transport points) for all organs and regulatory systems of the body shows the enormous influence of the bladder meridian on our body.

A disorder of the bladder meridian will initially show up in its key areas. There will be tension along its pathway, in the occiput, along the spine and on the back. When the power is permanently switched on, sleep will be superficial and restless, accompanied by increased sweating. The appetite suffers, the intestines are sensitive, as is the bladder. Blood pressure is off the scale, and cardiovascular disorders are on the horizon. It's the task of the life principle of the bladder meridian to recognise when it is necessary to curb the system. We also need to understand how much we ourselves contribute so that we experience stress as an exaggerated burden.

When the life principle of the bladder meridian is well developed, we have a sense of the limits of our physical and mental performance. We are able to manage ourselves excellently during times of strain. We are conscious of the necessity of breaks and recuperation. And we manage to flip the switch from sympathetic to parasympathetic mode. The latter then takes care of maintaining, recreating and building up the body's reserves. It slows down the pulse, lowers the blood pressure and stimulates the intestinal tract in order to process food and eliminate waste. The energy thus gained is offered to the body during deep and restorative sleep.

Of course, the pendulum can also swing too much towards the parasympathetic nervous system. Then we are constantly in the doldrums and find it impossible to become active. Body and mind are apathetic. What's lacking is strength, the willingness to fight for something or, if needed, to flee. A well-developed life principle of the bladder meridian allows us to adapt as much as possible to the prevailing challenges of life. The balance of yin and yang, as well as that of the sympathetic and parasympathetic nervous systems, is of crucial importance for our health so that everything can remain in flux.

SYMPTOMS ASSOCIATED WITH THE BLADDER MERIDIAN

Muscular tension, occipital pain, back pain, disturbed sleep, increased sweating, increased or reduced pulse rate, unstable blood pressure, high blood pressure, low blood pressure, tiredness, digestive disorders, irritable bowel syndrome, constipation, irritable bladder...

The Golden Stream

The bladder's task is wastewater disposal. Together with the kidneys, it forms the body's sewage plant and cleaning service, eliminating via the urine the filtered metabolic waste that is of no further use. As always in TCM, there is no differentiation between the physical and emotional aspects. The soul, too, creates waste that burdens the body. This refers mainly to emotions that threaten to flood us: emotions we are unable to process due to their intensity and which we should therefore get rid of as quickly as possible. Whenever there is too much pressure on the system, the bladder pays for it.

In this respect, the bladder meridian has an important regulatory function: it is considered an important protector of the heart, which tends to react very sensitively to highly intense emotions. The bladder meridian is the emperor's lightning conductor; it is the release valve protecting him from overload. The heart is not supposed to become too upset. If it does, the bladder responds by draining the emotional overflow via the urine. When we are scared to death or have a shock, we wet our pants. In the case of pronounced inner tension, we have to void our bladder several times per hour. However, the pressure often doesn't even have to be that severe or intense, and even minor stress can be sufficient to turn us into regulars on the toilet. The life principle of the bladder is indicative of how much psychological pressure we can stand and how we deal with it. The bladder meridian can be seen as a holding basin and the urine as the effluent of the soul.

When the bladder is full, it makes sense to empty it, simply letting go, letting it happen, before the water backs up. The same is true for the emotional realm. If the life principle of the bladder is well integrated, we're not afraid to give big emotion a free rein; we don't hold them back unnecessarily until they accumulate. We are able to cry when we are touched by something, angry when something annoys us, happy when something excites us. We go with the flow, as required by circumstances, like a little child allowing her feelings and her wee-wee to go their own free way. The difference is that a strong bladder meridian is able to consciously control and also to consciously relinquish control. It is able to manage its emotions.

An imbalanced bladder meridian, on the other hand, has problems with this kind of controlled loss of control, trying instead to contain its insecurity behind a massive dam. We try to pull ourselves together by hook or by crook, even if all we want to do is cry. We try to appear cool, even if that threatens to tear our heart apart. The fear of letting ourselves go is deep-seated. The free flow of emotions dries up, and they accumulate. They back up.

And all that despite the fact that an emotional outburst can be as liberating as completely voiding the bladder. A regular cleansing catharsis of the soul is necessary; otherwise, enormous inner tensions build up and a turbid pool of boiling soul water forms. The restrained emotions are bubbling under the surface but are unable to get out. On a physical level, we see urinary bladder infections. There is the burning desire to get rid of the inner pressure, but we're unable to achieve this. We are desperate to empty our bladder; nonetheless, only small amounts of urine are excreted, only dribbles, and even these come with considerable pain. We hold back what is urgent, what is burning. We hold it in the bladder and in the soul.

Another expression of a poorly developed life principle of the bladder meridian is the inability to restrain oneself at all. The bladder is weak and sensitive, and gets easily irritated. You are unable to withstand and deal with any emotional pressure. You weep easily; just a tiny push and everything flows, like a torrent, carrying you off against your will. And should things get too much emotionally, you simply piss off. A trivial midterm exam is enough to have you up at night ten times in order to relieve yourself. You have to leave important meetings like clockwork once an hour. A low stress tolerance coupled with poorly developed self-control may be indicators of an imbalanced bladder meridian.

All of the above are signs that it's about time to develop the bladder meridian's life principle. If it is strong, we're able stay emotionally with the flow, and we can even direct the flow according to requirements. We remain clear and focussed, and don't let ourselves be polluted or swept away by our emotions.

SYMPTOMS ASSOCIATED WITH THE BLADDER MERIDIAN

Cystitis, incontinence, increased or reduced desire to void one's bladder, urinary retention, weak pelvic floor, bedwetting...

The Bladder Meridian and the Psyche

Fight or Flight

The bladder meridian, with its close connection to the autonomic nervous system, not only controls our fight-or-flight mechanism on a physical level, but also endows us with the psychological capacity to fight for something or, depending on the situation, opt for flight. The life principle of the bladder meridian is needed when things get tight or we absolutely want to achieve something. However, the bladder meridian is not responsible for asking questions about the sense or non-sense of our actions, nor is it its task to align our aims with our inner values. Rather, its task is to provide us with the necessary fighting spirit. It bundles resources, willpower and the focus on the desired result; it gathers momentum; it prepares us for action. The bladder meridian knows that sometimes a compromise is quite simply not helpful; sometimes we just have to take the bull by the horns and stay on the ball, whatever the price. It's worth it to fight for our dreams. It's worth it to fight for the love of our life. These days, it's also much more common that we have to fight for our job. And when we are confronted with serious illnesses, it requires an extremely tenacious fighting spirit. In all these situations, the bladder meridian helps us to keep fighting with all our strength and all our might. It provides us with stamina and strong nerves. It doesn't let us down.

But a poorly developed life principle of the bladder meridian will, straight away, lose its nerves when confronted with big challenges or important goals. We prefer to run away rather than face something. We act and react based on insecurity and fear. At its worst, our whole life can deteriorate into being in constant flight mode. We give up, we give up on ourselves, before we have even properly begun with something. We're running away from every-day life, confrontations, closeness, our desires, our needs, from ourselves. At each and every opportunity, we energetically wet our pants. Or we freeze, losing our mobility. We change nothing, we don't do anything; we stick our head in the sand and hope that we are overlooked, and life will somehow smooth the waves for us. A weak bladder meridian results in being easily startled and having an extremely hesitant attitude. We live in denial of any problems and conflicts on our path until it becomes utterly unavoidable to tackle them.

Occasionally, however, it does make a lot of sense to take to one's heels and escape. In our dog-eat-dog society that relies on fight and denial, and where stress has become a fashion statement and burn-out a fashionable complaint, it is actually healthy to go for refuge, take some time out, make yourself scarce. A bladder meridian with a well-integrated life principle knows when enough is enough, and when the body needs a break. Simply leaving everything behind and disappearing off for a while: it's important to occasionally let things be as they are, to let the world keep turning. This is an attitude an imbalanced bladder meridian may neither believe in nor accept. It fights for fighting's sake. It turns us into a fighting machine that stops at nothing, focussed on its goal, regardless of the consequences, whatever the cost. Surrendering is not an option, even if it means surrendering yourself because it's no longer you holding the rudder but a crazed bladder meridian. Such people see everything as a sport, everything as a competition, everyone a rival. For them, it's paramount to win. There is, of course, a direct correlation with self-esteem and self-affirmation. If you slow down, you lose. It's therefore not possible to relax, not even for a minute. Flexibility is also lost along the way. You constantly try to force the river of life instead of giving yourself up to it and drifting along with it.

A bladder meridian with a well-developed life principle knows when the time is right for a fight and when it's time to walk away. And it knows that to flee from certain things is often the only sensible response since everything else would only consume vast amounts of time and energy. This insight leads to confident equanimity that allows you to take things as they come.

Resistance to Stress, Resilience and Equanimity

The development and integration of the bladder meridian can be recognised by how we deal with stress. Stress can be considered a subjective sensation indicating that one's resources are in short supply or not sufficient to cope with a particular situation. This sensation strongly depends on individual perception and the evaluation of the challenge. What can take one person to their limits is considered an exciting challenge by another. A robust bladder meridian will overcome even the biggest hurdles; it stands for high stress resistance – such people are tough and don't easily break down under pressure. They go with the flow. They are able to self-regulate according to requirements. They accelerate as needed and relax when possible. Stress symptoms are triggered either not at all or only at a later stage because they don't feel as if they're being helplessly subjected to the cause of stress. They are resilient.

Resilience describes the ability of a material or substance to return to its original shape after external interference. The term is based on the Latin *resilire*, which means 'to recoil, to rebound'. Resilience provides us with the capacity to deal constructively with disturbances, disruptions or change. Resilience allows us to stay healthy or develop even greater strength despite severe strain or adverse life events. A well-developed life principle of the bladder meridian manifests in a high capacity for resilience as it is able to govern and control the necessary traits, including the entire range from willpower to a fighting spirit, and also quick recuperation.

In contrast, a weak bladder meridian easily reacts in an exaggerated manner when stress raises its head. Even minor issues lead to upset, and feelings of being overwhelmed will set in quickly. The threshold for frustration is low. It's difficult to tolerate any form of stress. Our emotional state is anything but stable and balanced. We tilt at windmills and run away from mice. We are quick to throw in the towel. We are faint-hearted. Accordingly, we are easily irritated, nervous, restless – in a nutshell: we are easily stressed. Once triggered, we are stuck with the stress; it breathes down our neck and won't let go, even once the causative circumstances have long since changed. We are in a tense state around the clock. We have lost the ability to return spontaneously to our original form. We are the opposite of resilient: we're not good at coping.

For modern-day living, it is crucial to have a bladder meridian with a well-developed life principle. In times that are getting increasingly faster, more challenging and ever more uncertain, a high stress tolerance coupled with good resilience is essential for staying balanced.

Signs of an Imbalanced and Balanced Bladder Meridian

Signs of an Imbalanced Bladder Meridian

- Tendency to hyperactivity or apathy
- Getting easily stressed or worked up, quickly overwhelmed
- Quick to lose one's nerve, unable to meet a challenge
- Tendency to a nervous bladder, urgency during the night, cystitis...
- Difficulty relaxing, calming down and recuperating
- Prone to crying or weeping; finding it difficult to hold back or admit emotions

Signs of a Balanced Bladder Meridian

- Ability to work under pressure, high stress tolerance
- Adapting to demands while having the capacity for staying calm
- Good fighting spirit coupled with nerves of steel
- High resilience
- Able to show emotions and admit to weaknesses

How to Strengthen the Life Principle of the Bladder Meridian

Increasing Stress Tolerance

If you would like to strengthen the life principle of the bladder meridian, it is of benefit to work on your stress tolerance. Unfortunately, there is no key that can simply open the gate to more equanimity. Rather, an increase in your stress tolerance is the result of several factors coming together. Give yourself about two weeks to lay a foundation. The following measures have proven very successful. Set priorities! This may sound mundane but, followed through consistently, it's a very helpful strategy. Separate what's important from what isn't. Reduce what's important by 50%. Once you've done this, enjoy a break! This, too, is extremely important. The best way to spend your break is with breathing exercises in the form of a short meditation. The breath calms the body, and the meditation calms the mind. Try to sleep more during those two weeks. Extending your regular sleeping hours by only 30 minutes will make quite a difference. And if you're unable to sleep during that extra time, simply stay in bed. Once again, use the time for breathing and meditating. Another part of the programme is yoga: practise yoga every other day. Yoga is excellent for balancing the autonomic nervous system. And last but not least, when the going gets tough, don't be shy about asking for help and support. Of course, there are a lot of other things for increasing one's stress tolerance and resilience. To begin with, really take yourself and your needs seriously for once, and pursue whatever you enjoy most for a couple of weeks. Your bladder meridian will be very grateful.

Have a Cry

A Jewish adage says, 'What soap is for the body, tears are for the soul.' This, too, expresses the cleansing aspect of the bladder meridian. We cry whenever our emotions threaten to flood us, whether it's grief, joy, pain or anger. Simply do it! Make use of the next opportunity and let your feelings flow freely. You will see how good that feels – and you will also see how, despite having a cry, the world keeps on turning. Every emotional outburst can stabilise and balance our emotions by resolving emotional tension. To show emotions is, after all, also a sign of strength. If crying doesn't work out, remember that each feeling is right and of sufficient value to be shown. Stay with the flow!

The Pathway of the Bladder Meridian

The bladder meridian arises in a depression slightly above the inner corner of the eye at the point Bladder 1. It continues towards the inner end of the eyebrow, the location of Bladder 2. From there, it travels straight upwards over the forehead to just beyond the hair-line, where, at Bladder 3, it changes course slightly, moving about one and a half thumb-widths in a lateral direction to Bladder 4. From Bladder 4, the meridian runs parallel to the midline over the head and the occiput to reach Bladder 10, situated at the insertion of the trapezius at the back of the head, slightly less than one and a half thumb-widths from the midline. Here, at Bladder 10, the meridian divides into two branches.

The inner branch travels from Bladder 10 laterally to Bladder 11, located one and a half thumb-widths from the midline of the back, level with the spinous process of the first thoracic vertebra. From there, it descends the back in a straight line one and a half thumb-widths parallel to the midline to Bladder 30, which is level with the fourth sacral foramen. At this point the meridian switches back upwards to Bladder 31, located directly in the first sacral foramen. The bladder meridian now continues downwards again, following the sacral foramina and then the coccyx (tailbone), where it begins to curve outwards in the direction of the gluteal fold. The next important landmark is Bladder 36, located below the ischial tuberosity at the midpoint of the gluteal fold. From Bladder 36, the bladder meridian runs between two clearly palpable muscle bellies (biceps femoris and semitendinosus) along the middle of the back of the thigh to reach the knee crease, where it veers slightly outward to Bladder 39, located on the outer edge of the knee crease. From there it continues to the midpoint of the knee crease, where Bladder 40 can be found. This is also the point where the outer and inner branches merge again.

The outer branch of the bladder meridian curves outward from Bladder 10 to Bladder 41, located three thumb-widths lateral to the midline and level with the second thoracic vertebra. From Bladder 41, the bladder meridian descends the back in a straight line, running three thumb-widths parallel to the midline, to reach Bladder 54, located at the level of Bladder 30. The outer branch now curves in a gentle arc to Bladder 40.

Having passed the knee crease, the bladder meridian runs between the two heads of gastrocnemius. At the lower end of the two heads is the point Bladder 57. The meridian continues to follow the outer edge of gastrocnemius. It then moves further laterally and, as it emerges from the calf musculature, runs alongside the Achilles tendon to Bladder 60, midway between this tendon and the lateral malleolus. A depression approximately one and half thumb-widths perpendicularly below Bladder 60 is the location of Bladder 61. The bladder meridian then slightly descends again to reach Bladder 62 on the lower border of the lateral malleolus. From there, the meridian continues to Bladder 63, which can be found in a depression on the outer edge of the foot, directly past the calcaneus (heel bone). The meridian further follows the outer edge of the foot, on the border of the dorsal and plantar aspects passing Bladder 64 (just distal to the joint of the fifth metatarsal bone) until it reaches its final point, Bladder 67, on the outer corner of the small toe.

Key Areas of the Bladder Meridian

Head and Occiput

The bladder meridian begins above the inner corner of the eye at the point Bladder 1, *jing ming* or 'Bright Eyes'. Bladder 1 has a direct connection to the tear glands, indicating the relationship between the bladder meridian and the free flow of our emotions. The free flow of the bladder meridian manifests, in turn, in the occiput. This is where stress tends to become entrenched. Very tense or painful occipital musculature is often the result of sitting for too long in conjunction with much strain and pressure or extreme tiredness. Directly at the transition from the head to the spine, at the lower border of the occiput, we find Bladder 10, *tian zhu* or 'Celestial Pillar'. The cervical spine can be seen as a pillar supporting heaven. However, stress and strain can lead to the head becoming disengaged from the body. When stress is severe, we are no longer aware of our needs, we suppress tiredness and discomfort, and we don't feel ourselves anymore. Body and mind are separated, the area around Bladder 10 is rock-hard, and everything stagnates in the head. With Bladder 10, we can re-open the connection and re-establish the relationship with heaven.

Back

The entire back is strongly controlled by the bladder meridian. The back is also the area where its correspondence with the autonomic nervous system, starting from the central spinous canal and innervating the entire body, shows up most. It's therefore not surprising that we find acupuncture points supporting all organ systems (so-called back-*shu* points) in precisely this section of the meridian. This shows that an imbalance in the autonomic nervous system may have an influence on the entire body and can be the cause of many disorders, on both a physical and mental level. There are 40 acupuncture points in total in this section of the bladder meridian. No other meridian has such a high concentration of points in one area.

Furthermore, the back mirrors how we deal with stress and tension. It shows whether we easily end up with our back to the wall since we're lacking the necessary backbone to keep an upright posture. It's a sign that the life principle of the bladder meridian does not provide the necessary balance when we're overwhelmed, and the pressure we're under may break our spine. Or we bend over backwards just for the possibility of a little pat on the back. A harmonious bladder energy, on the other hand, provides us with a propitious tailwind and a strong and broad back that insults and criticisms roll off like water off a duck's back – meaning we don't care what others think of us and we're not going to break our back for the whims of others. The bladder meridian keeps our backs straight and free. After all, the entire back is sensitive to disorders in the bladder meridian, and TCM treats most back pain directly through the bladder meridian.

The Bladder Meridian: Key Points

- Associated element: Water element
- Quality: Yang
- Time on the organ clock: 3pm–5pm
- Animal quality: Monkey
- Partner meridian: Kidney meridian
- Twinned meridian: Small intestine meridian
- Opposite meridian: Lung meridian

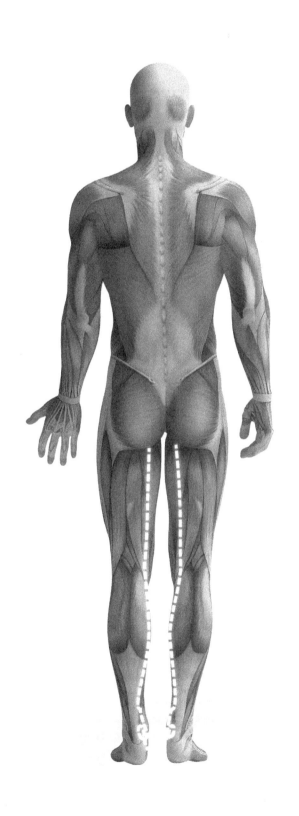

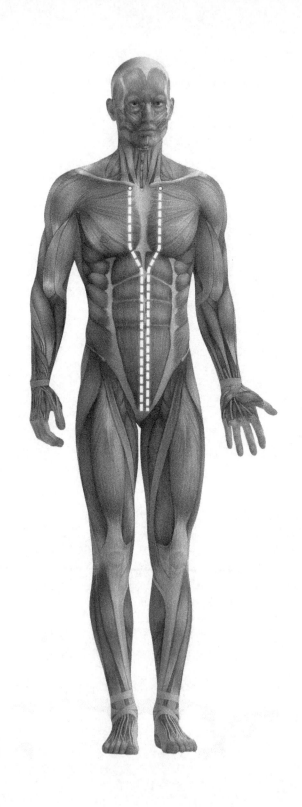

Chapter 11

The Kidney Meridian

Fulfilling Your Potential

Questions for the Kidney Meridian

- Do I know precisely what my strengths and weaknesses are?
- Do I know who I am and what I want?
- Do I have sufficient self-confidence?
- Do I feel I am of value?
- Do I have the courage to leave my comfort zone?
- Am I able to take risks?
- Do I have much willpower and drive?
- Do I have basic trust?
- Do I trust others?
- Do I often doubt myself?
- Do I often feel insecure and anxious?

The Life Principle of the Kidney Meridian

Why am I here? What is my purpose on this planet? What is my mission? Big questions requiring big answers. The life principle of the kidney meridian provides those answers: it gets to the bottom of things; it passionately and thoroughly investigates, until it knows what's really going on, especially if it's about our potential and the possibilities for development that go along with it. TCM likes to compare the kidneys to a seed. The seed contains all the information that is necessary for the plant to fully evolve, whether it's a daisy or a palm tree. The crucial factor is what kind of seed you are, since for every seed there are better and worse habitats. Sown on a hot, sandy tropical beach, a daisy would hardly evolve according to its potential; nor would a palm tree in Siberia. Nature cleverly regulates this, compensating for wrong choices.

In our lives, that's not always so easy. Whether it affects our job, our relationships or our leisure time, the potential slumbering deep within us isn't always realised, because we're in the wrong place at the wrong time, because of wrong conditions and wrong plans. But the life principle of the kidneys knows precisely what is slumbering within. It knows what is needed to make the most of it. It has at its disposal the strength, the courage and the will to implement the relevant measures, and the tenacity to pursue them. It answers the questions that get to the core of what life is about: Who am I? What do I want? How can I reach my goals?

Every person has strengths, talents and aptitudes. Often, these already manifest in early childhood, which is also the time when the life principle of the kidneys begins to develop. It's the time when it can be promoted or inhibited. When children get the necessary attention, affection and recognition by their caregivers, they feel that they and their abilities are seen. They feel encouraged and learn to trust their abilities. This provides safety, so much so that over time healthy self-confidence will build up: the foundation to stand powerfully on your own feet later on, to stand up for yourself and your potential. Precisely for this reason, the pathway of the kidney meridian begins at the feet.

Self-confidence is an essential aspect of the kidney meridian and the foundation for further qualities closely associated with the kidneys. If we trust ourselves, we will be more courageous. If we trust ourselves, we dare to do things, take risks, venture into uncertain realms. We have and show our courage. We'll jump in at the deep end because we know that we can swim and won't drown. Self-confidence is a crucially important quality if you want to unleash your full potential. You need to be true to yourself when there is a headwind or you're entering unknown territory. Fear won't take you very far. Because angst and fear paralyse. 'Angst' derives from the Indo-Germanic *anghu* meaning 'restrictive'. Angst restricts; it crushes dreams, hopes, longings and desires. Fear gives rise to doubt, in particular about yourself. Fear, insecurity and self-doubt are an expression of kidneys with a poorly developed life principle. Fear and doubt are two profoundly inhibiting factors for growth and development. Besides courage, these processes also require great willpower. This, too, is rooted in the kidneys, and it will stand on shaky legs when constant doubts pull the rug from under its feet.

Willpower is the ability to govern yourself. If you are able to utilise your willpower properly, you will be able to mobilise yourself, strive towards goals that are important to you and, with tenacity, eventually reach them. You're able to achieve things. You achieve self-efficacy and self-determination. Confidence, courage and willpower allow you to cope with even the biggest challenges. You can live your destiny. If you don't, you will be controlled – by life, by other people, by coincidences, by fate. Instead of acting, you're only reacting. You become the palm tree planted in Siberia against its will; your developmental chances are zero. Weakness instead of strength governs the life principle of the kidneys – a far cry from being the person you could be.

The Kidney Meridian and the Body

Having a Point and Seeing it Through

The kidney meridian begins at the feet. It takes courage and will-power to stand on your own two feet. But it's the only way to get a foothold in what matches our potential. A mission that matches our true nature, our personality, our abilities and our talents until we finally stand on familiar ground, able to master the challenges of life with ease. Light-footed and without much effort, with the personal profile of a relaxed pro. We're competent, confident, expe-rienced. There's no trace of insecurity, not a whiff of self-doubt. This allows you to live generously since you appreciate your worth and won't sell yourself short. And high self-esteem makes for a high market value, professionally, in your relationships and for your general position in life. Just as a tree in the right place and the right climate can produce an excellent yield, so does a strong kidney meridian provide abundance in all areas of life. External abundance is always an expression of internal abundance, which arises by doing and embodying what is a true expression of yourself. It occurs naturally when you follow yourself.

The feet can be seen as the roots of the body. With our feet, we take up our position; our feet also root us in our existence. Strong ankles provide stability. Good circulation in the feet brings about liveliness, warmth and instinct. We know where we stand in life. Firm and deep roots nourish not only our confidence but also our basic trust and gut feeling. Basic trust means to be able to trust others and the world, not blindly, but with awareness. This results in an optimistic and solution-oriented attitude, which is indispensable for fully and thoroughly committing to something, whether it's long-term goals in your profession or your relationship. You're happy to go 'all in' at any time: the capacity for strong commitment is an expression of a strong kidney meridian. You're not afraid to devote yourself to something with your heart and soul, because this kind of dedication can't be equated with throwing yourself on someone's mercy. Rather, it's an expression and an act of your conscious free will. Nonetheless, should you stumble at some point, you will have sufficient self-assurance to land on your feet again.

However, if the life principle of the kidneys is only poorly developed, there is the danger of tripping yourself up again and again because you get cold feet far too quickly when an exciting challenge knocks on the door. Due to your insecurity, you prefer to tread water instead of getting underway, pursuing your goals and exploiting your opportunities. Or you easily buckle under stress because owing to your weak roots there is no steadfastness. You're not very resilient, so you like to avoid any bigger tasks. There is little willingness to jump in at the deep end. You prefer to have a warm shower in the comfort of your home. In a worst-case scenario, a subtle but constantly present fear of life, fed by serious self-doubt, dominates. There is fear of emotions, which, in TCM, is directly correlated with the kidneys. There is no phobia without a link to the kidneys, whether it's ablutophobia (fear of washing/bathing), or zemmiphobia (fear of naked mole rats).

The tendency towards instability also manifests in the further pathway of the kidney meridian, especially at the knees. The impending threat to leave our comfort zone makes our knees weak and shaky. A weak kidney meridian may easily force us on to our knees or to succumb to the will of others. Because we don't have a firm standpoint, it's easy to be manipulated. Unable to provide stability for ourselves, we prefer to hold on to others. This provides safety and guidance. But it also leads to fear of loss, jealousy and holding on because we are scared to lose the other person or ourselves. This can result in excessive clinginess, especially in relationships. To avoid risk at all costs, we're even prepared to let ourselves be trampled underfoot. We're a far cry from the person we could be.

Weak roots and a weak trunk can be the substrate for many problems in all areas influenced by the kidney meridian, such as sensitive cold feet, oedema, unstable ankles or chronic knee problems. Conversely, a well-developed life principle of the kidneys provides strength and energy in precisely these areas of the body, along with the emotional correspondences. We know where we stand in life, what we want. We have the strength to be true to ourselves.

SYMPTOMS ASSOCIATED WITH THE KIDNEY MERIDIAN

Cold feet, sweaty feet, overly sensitive feet, unstable ankles, unstable knees, many forms of knee problems, oedema around the ankles and knees, anxiety disorders...

The Ravages of Time

Back to the seed: the kidneys store our entire potential. TCM refers to this as the essence or *jing*. The essence is our fuel, our super petrol, our life energy. When our *jing* is used up, we die. For this reason, TCM and the approach to health of many Asian philosophies are particularly concerned with maintaining and cultivating the *jing*. You could imagine the kidneys as a bank account and the essence as your seed money. If endowed with a few million in *jing* from the start, you can afford a lot, live unhealthily and indulge in a wide range of excesses. You have vitality and reserves without having to take much care of them. These are precisely the people who are often held up as evidence that it is perfectly possible to grow old despite burning the candle at both ends. We should be grateful to our parents for having filled our *jing* account with such a surplus. Strong and healthy parents, young at the time of conception and at the pinnacle of their strength, provide the ideal prerequisites for an account with a satisfying balance in the kidneys.

Western science refers to this scenario as the power of the genes. It means much the same thing, including that lifestyle influences the outcome. People who are equipped with only a smaller starter kit have to be better at budgeting or they need to earn more. They can do this by means of a sensible diet, regular exercise, a relaxed mental attitude and, in particular, activities that are fulfilling. That way, they use up less energy so that it's not necessary to rely too much on their essence. A frugal lifestyle saves and protects from premature bankruptcy. These are people who have to be more careful about their health.

No matter whether there is much or little essence, public enemy number one is stress caused by insecurity. For the kidneys, even a minor lack of confidence can result in constantly present insecurity. You're unsure about yourself. Plagued by doubts, your everyday life turns into a highly stressful affair. Stress turns primarily to the bladder meridian, which, when activated, drains energy from the kidney meridian: fight-or-flight mode. We're tense, even too tense, and overwhelmed. The stress hormone levels gradually rise. This gnaws away at our essence. What the ancient Chinese already knew more than two thousand years ago is now also considered common sense by science: long-term intense stress weakens the body and the immune system. Stress accelerates ageing, as does an excessive lifestyle, overdosing on pleasures of any kind, be it overeating, boozing, taking drugs or sex. All this devours energy, as do serious illnesses and other existential crises. And the kidneys, as administrators of the essence, control all the areas in the body where physical decline may become apparent.

Our teeth and hair are particularly sensitive substances. Both are a favourite haunt of the ravages of time. The condition of our teeth has always been a gauge as to whether we're physically worthy of credit. And many people may have first-hand experience that intense stress can result in hair loss or turn it grey. However, it's perfectly normal in old age, when the balance of the kidneys' account is waning, that these symbols of energy and strength will lose their vitality. But when stress, excesses or crises devour the essence, this process can begin much earlier.

What else abandons us as we age? Our ears, which in TCM are considered the mirror image of the kidneys. Thus, in statues of the Buddha, the ears are often depicted as almost elephant-like in size, an expression of an abundance of essence and potential. And ears react very sensitively to stress. Tinnitus, sudden deafness or hearing loss often occur during periods of intense stress and are an expression of a weakening of the kidney energy. Weak kidneys also have an impact on fertility since the reproductive organs are directly controlled by the kidney meridian, which, if lacking in energy, is unable to optimally supply the lower abdomen. This results in infertility, impotence, early menopause or loss of libido. The pelvic floor in general reflects the strength of the kidney meridian, and it will begin to weaken when the essence is dwindling. It won't close properly any more, with symptoms ranging from mild dribbling to severe incontinence.

And last but not least, it's the turn of our brain and bones. With the essence in decline, the bones lose their density and the brain sustains a loss of performance. Osteoporosis, sometimes with onset before the age of 30, memory loss, forgetfulness. The capacity and functionality of our grey matter is shrinking. Conversely, treating our kidney essence well will lead to good physical vitality, even at an advanced age. There are certainly people in their seventies or eighties who still have all their teeth and hair and a strong libido, and who appear biologically much younger than their actual age. However, if, due to an unfortunate lifestyle, we have squandered our essence too early, then we will appear much older than we are according to our birth certificate: live fast, die young.

The kidneys, as the store of the essence, have a strong influence on our entire body. The best way of preserving and cultivating our energy is by looking at what the life principle of the kidneys wants to teach us: to live our full potential. Of course, diet, exercise, yoga and meditation are all very useful. However, once you have found your place in life that is right for you, provides you with positive challenges and allows you to make the most of who you are, then you will be in a continuous state of flow, and if you're in flow, you need less energy. Often, you may even get more energy back than you have invested. But in a state of anti-flow, there will be friction on all levels. This drains energy. It doesn't keep you young. It makes you age before your time.

Fatigue, premature ageing, teeth problems, hair loss, premature greying of hair, memory problems, tinnitus, sudden deafness, hearing loss, problems with bone density, infertility, early menopause, impotence, lack of libido, incontinence...

The Kidney Meridian and the Psyche

Authenticity, Autonomy and Relationships

When the life principle of your kidneys is well developed, you are, more than anything else, authentic. You know who you are, and you know what you are. You know yourself. You accept and embrace yourself, with all your strengths and weaknesses, all your shortcomings and all your talents. You therefore don't have to play-act; you don't need to pretend or dissemble. You can afford to leave the game of superficiality and mask-wearing behind. You do what you need to do, you live your life; you're at peace with yourself, whatever others may think about you. This leads to credibility and sincerity, which also manifests in your posture. You have a straight spine; you're certainly not spineless – you can back yourself up. In TCM, the kidney meridian also supports the spine. If we are insecure and full of self-doubt, we tend to bend over backwards and be subservient in order to please others and to make sure our head is kept below the parapet. We pretend to be something we are not, because we fear not being accepted, being caught up in a conflict or arousing opposition. Rather, we genuflect before both ourselves and life – a weakness in the life principle of our kidney meridian.

Authentic people express their views clearly and directly because they don't depend on the confirmation of others. They call a spade a spade without attributing any value to it. They have an opinion and stand by it without getting cold feet. A strongly evolved kidney meridian doesn't require pretentiousness or showmanship. It can afford to be simple and natural. It follows its path with the aim of realising its potential. This path can take it to the limits of rules and norms. Should societal conventions get in the way of their development, assertive kidneys will remain on course, owing to their strength to weather difficulties. Rather than following trends, the opinions of others, or temporary fads, they remain true to their principles.

This makes them trendsetters, pioneers, trailblazers, role models. It all leads to a high degree of autonomy and sovereignty. A well-integrated life principle of the kidney meridian ensures that you can be happy in your own company, that you don't need others in order to define yourself. You'd much rather have few but deep and meaningful friendships. Conversely, a weak life principle of the kidneys will result in constantly requiring validation by others, since you're not standing on your own two feet. This can lead to a variety of problems, especially regarding intimate relationships, which have a lot of kidney involvement. After all, the kidneys are a paired organ. And the kidney meridian governs all reproductive processes, including sexuality.

The more you manage to fulfil your potential, the more complete you become as a person. If we don't actually live our lives, we tend to project on to others what is lying dormant within us. They may complement what we are missing. A poorly developed life principle of the kidneys has a propensity to look for a person who can provide these additions. This can quickly result in us 'needing' this person because otherwise we'd be 'missing' something. And if at some point we are really missing something, then we have 'lost' it. This 'it' would be ourselves. The fear of loss of self can cause us to sell our soul, to present ourselves as a daisy even though we are a palm tree. Authenticity and autonomy are sacrificed on the altar of compromise. However, if we were to live our life like that, we would wither rather than blossom. It would be the surest way into a form of dependency that, in the long run, would be hardly constructive.

The life principle of the kidneys knows that what we have realised in ourselves cannot be taken from us. Self-actualisation is the foundation for freedom in life and in relationships.

Motivation, Willpower and Money

In TCM, motivation and willpower have a close connection with the kidneys. Strong kidneys, strong motivation, strong willpower – that's certainly the case. But it is about more than that. It's about the right motivation. One's motivation harbours one's motives. If we have an inner vision that we want to set our course for, we will be motivated, we will persevere, we want to succeed. The clearer our inner vision, the greater the resulting driving force. The life principle of the kidneys represents our potential, our possibilities, our talents. It stands for our inner values, for what we consider truly important in our lives. Motivation built on our inner values and our potential has meaning. If we encounter any challenges, we're happy to deal with them for their own sake, because we know they are right and because they will lead us to our destination. The result is an extraordinarily strong motivation arising from the core of our nature, in turn leading to a matching drive and willpower.

This includes the ability to be clear about our long-term goals without getting bogged down by minor details or background noise. A well-integrated life principle of the kidneys knows which path to take, and even if some junctions may appear very exciting, we can resist the temptation to turn off or take a break. We are able to subordinate short-term pleasures to long-term contentment. This, too, can be considered a sign of strong willpower, the capacity to postpone the fulfilment of needs as an intelligent way of dealing with our resources. A strong kidney meridian knows how to budget wisely and will invest its energy where, in the long run, the highest returns can be expected, not only in the form of fulfilment and contentment but also in terms of money and capital. People with a strong kidney meridian tend to accumulate rather than scatter. They have the capacity to become wealthy, both internally and externally.

A weakness in the life principle of the kidney meridian will therefore have profound effects on a person's life. If you don't know where you're going, you may likely arrive nowhere, or you may end up where the wind of life blew you. Distractions are always welcome. Quick gratification instead of a comprehensive masterplan. What needs to be done will most likely get postponed – procrastination at world championship level. Nonetheless, should goals appear on the horizon, you will find it difficult to pursue them. And whyever should you? Of course, there could be some external motivation: doing things for a reward or to avoid punishment. If either of those stimuli is strong enough, even people with weak kidneys will get going. But they have to fight hard as their willpower lacks the necessary foundation. This consumes a lot of energy so that such attempts tend to be short-lived. Bigger challenges often end up with sore feet. One is well on the way towards burnout.

And what's more, by being externally motivated, you may be pursuing goals which you don't really want to reach, and which have little to do with your inner values. If the life principle of the kidneys is weak, you will be especially susceptible to this kind of situation as deep insecurity makes you want to please others. But even if such people-pleasing behaviour leads to success and wealth, an inner emptiness will remain because your actions are devoid of a deeper meaning.

For the life principle of the kidneys, it is therefore important to take some time out now and again and to reflect on some clear questions: Where do I stand at this moment in time? Where do I want to be? Why do I want to be there? Am I still pursuing the right goals? And are my goals in line with my potential and my abilities? If there are clear answers to these questions, you're on the right path to living the life principle of the kidneys.

Signs of an Imbalanced and Balanced Kidney Meridian

Signs of an Imbalanced Kidney Meridian

- Little self-confidence, little self-esteem, little self-awareness
- Insecurity, self-doubt, much anxiety
- Little drive and stamina, little willpower
- Weak feet, knees and legs, sensitivity to cold
- Little energy, premature ageing
- Tendency to feel overwhelmed, risk of burnout

Signs of a Balanced Kidney Meridian

- Natural self-confidence and authenticity
- Healthy courage and a high degree of confidence in self
- Highly autonomous, independent and self-sufficient
- Strong willpower, good stamina, dynamic drive
- High energy levels and strong physical resources
- Good at dealing with money and assets
- Evolving and growing are part of the processes of life

How to Strengthen the Life Principle of the Kidney Meridian

Who Am I? What Defines Me?

Getting to the bottom of the kidney's life principle requires regular time out for reflecting and taking stock. To that end, dedicate a weekend to yourself at least twice a year. Who we really are is probably one of the most crucial philosophical questions. So perhaps the question should be modified to: What can I do really well? What hidden talents are slumbering deep inside me? What is it that I have wanted to do all my life? What is important to me in life? What are my deepest inner values? And if you were a cartoon hero, what would be your superpower? Correlate your answers to these questions with your current situation: Where am I right now? Are the goals I'm pursuing still relevant? Do they bring me closer to my true self? Or am I getting further and further away from who I really am? Write your answers down by hand. And never be afraid of changing course. Just do it!

Jumping in at the Deep End

Once a week, with full awareness, jump in at the deep end! Do something that would normally give you cold feet. Face the challenges that make your knees tremble a bit. Do something out of the ordinary! Go climbing. Speak to a complete stranger in the street. Book a holiday on impulse. Run naked through the rain. What's important: ideally choose a level of difficulty promising failure or success in equal measure. It's not about success. It's about the effort you have to muster.

The Pathway of the Kidney Meridian

The kidney meridian begins at Kidney 1, in a depression on the sole of the foot located between the base joints of the second and third metatarsal bones. It courses along the sole of the foot towards the heel and then veers medially towards the arch of the foot. At the highest point of the arch (anterior and inferior to the border of the navicular bone) is Kidney 2. From there the meridian travels to Kidney 3, located at the midpoint of a line connecting the Achilles tendon and the medial malleolus. The meridian then curves downwards to Kidney 4 (at the inner border of the Achilles tendon attachment), on to Kidney 5 (a thumb-width below Kidney 3) and to Kidney 6 (directly below the medial malleolus).

From Kidney 6, the kidney meridian courses via Kidney 7 (three thumb-widths above Kidney 3) towards Spleen 6 (three thumb-widths above the medial malleolus, on the posterior border of the tibia). This is the meeting point of the three yin meridians of the leg (liver, spleen, kidneys). The kidney meridian then ascends along the medial aspect of the two-headed gastrocnemius to Kidney 10, which is located on the medial border of the knee crease, between the tendons of the semitendinosus and the semimembranosus. The kidney meridian continues between these two muscles, close to the femur, towards the pelvis and the buttock musculature, where, at the gluteal fold, it disappears into the interior of the body, encircling the genitals as it does so.

The kidney meridian re-emerges on the anterior aspect of the body, at the upper border of the pubic symphysis, approximately half a thumb-width lateral to the midline, and continues to ascend vertically at this distance towards the costal arch. An important point, Kidney 16, can be found at the level of the navel. Just inferior to the costal arch, the kidney meridian curves diagonally in a lateral direction, traversing the costal arch. It then travels at a distance of about two thumb-widths lateral to the midline alongside the breast bone upwards towards the collarbone. The terminal point, Kidney 27, is located two thumb-widths lateral to the anterior midline, between the first rib and the clavicle.

Key Areas of the Kidney Meridian

Feet and Knees

The kidney meridian begins on the sole of the foot at Kidney 1 'Gushing Spring' or *yong quan*. If we truly stand on our own two feet, contributing with our potential to the world and living our destiny, we become like a gushing spring that draws from itself. We are well supplied with energy and can thus become a source of inspiration for others. Through Kidney 1 and the connection to the ground, we also connect with something bigger, with the supportive and sustaining quality of the earth. This engenders a basic and fundamental trust. We don't have to endure everything on our own; we can count on resources. Life becomes a gushing spring that supports us and catches us should we trip over our own feet or those of others. However, if the area around Kidney 1 is only poorly developed, we're lacking purchase, and our rootedness will be suboptimal. A plant with weak roots can't draw much water from the soil. It will wither, it won't blossom, it won't fulfil its destiny. This can also happen to humans. In that case, we're the opposite of a gushing spring and we won't turn into a powerful, stable river coming from the mountains and flowing towards the ocean.

This quality manifests particularly clearly at the point Kidney 3, the 'Great Ravine' or *tai xi*, which is located between the medial malleolus and the Achilles tendon. The stronger the ankles, the greater our steadfastness when acting for ourselves. Poorly developed ankles, on the other hand, can easily buckle under strain. Kidney 3 is a sensitive point. The Greek hero Achilles had only one vulnerable area on his entire body, and this was precisely the spot where he was hit. It is worth noting that the area around the ankle has a marked concentration of kidney points. Of the ten leg points of the kidney meridian, the first seven can be found in the section covering the foot and the ankle.

A further key point for steadfastness, Kidney 10, 'Yin Valley' or *yin gu*, is located at the knee. This area, too, raises the question: Do our knees easily buckle when faced with a challenge? Or are we able to push through the greatest difficulties without losing our footing?

Chest

Of the 27 points on the kidney meridian, seven are located on the foot and 17 on the anterior aspect of the torso. The message is clear: if we are true to ourselves, we can show ourselves just as we are. Without fear, with confidence in ourselves and our abilities. We don't have to protect our chest and belly, we don't have to hide; we're able to open up, we're able to cope with confrontations. A confident and upright yet flexible and lively posture is a good indicator of a well-integrated life principle of the kidney meridian. Being proud is allowed. Pride is the feeling of great contentment with oneself; it is an expression of self-esteem. Pride is like the joy that is rooted in the certainty of being special. And isn't every human being special? Along with the evolving of our potential grows our awareness of the unique nature of every individual being. It's okay and even right to show this – and where better than along the kidney meridian on the torso.

The Kidney Meridian: Key Points

- Associated element: Water element
- Quality: Yin
- Time on the organ clock: 5pm–7pm
- Animal quality: Rooster
- Partner meridian: Bladder meridian
- Twinned meridian: Heart meridian
- Opposite meridian: Large intestine meridian

Chapter 12

The Second Meridian Family: Heart, Small Intestine, Bladder and Kidneys

Individuation

According to the organ clock, the second meridian family begins with the heart (11am to 1pm), followed by the small intestine (1pm to 3pm), the bladder (3pm to 5pm) and the kidneys (5pm to 7pm). When the first meridian family has sufficiently matured so that basic needs and the ability for survival are secured, it is succeeded by the next big stage of childhood development, the step from infant to toddler. This step generally occurs around the twelfth month, with many of its characteristic abilities already beginning to evolve at six months – for example, exploring space through crawling, or playing with sounds as a precursor to language development. During this time of major change, the little person begins to distinguish increasingly between them and their environment. It's the awakening of the energies of the heart and small intestine. The *shen*, our conscious perception, becomes active. The small intestine meridian begins to separate, to discern. It informs the *shen* that there is an 'I' and other people, that there are subjects and objects. Both meridians and their respective range of functions are instrumental in the development of consciousness of self. At about 15 months, infants are able to recognise themselves in a mirror. At the same time, their vocabulary and their ability to articulate expand rapidly. Initially, there is an increase in naming objects. The small intestine recognises the diversity of things; the heart expresses this through language. This is followed by naming activities until even words such as 'you' and 'I' are used in the correct context.

At the same time, the increased desire for movement is clearly noticeable. Even if the baby may have been crawling or even standing previously, the energetic change from the first to the second meridian family is the decisive breakthrough towards toddlers taking their first steps. This is the responsibility of the bladder meridian. It begins at the eyes and terminates at the toes. It connects the entire posterior aspect of the body to form a unified whole and it facilitates forward movement. Forward movement in space is important as it fosters the feeling of being an independent individual on two independent legs. The consistent feedback of sensory stimuli as well as experiencing autonomous and aware movement in space promotes the toddler's development of identity. The maturing identity is then joined by the kidney meridian, along with the discovery of one's own free will. It's for a reason that this phase is referred to as the autonomy stage. It is the beginning of the defiant stage: defiance as the manifestation of the child's desire to express his or her personality. The establishment of the self and the discovery of its abilities represents the central task of the second meridian family, with the core questions being: Who am I? What do I want? How can I accomplish my goals? The second meridian family relates predominantly to the fourth level of Maslow's hierarchy of needs, which is concerned with the needs of the individual.

Once again, it requires much care and devotion to support this developmental stage. Toddlers will be oscillating between exploring their environment and returning to safety and comfort. The increase in autonomy represents a state of conflicting priorities, with desire for more independence while still needing much help. It is part and parcel of every growth process to overcome fears; it's like entering uncharted territory. The central topic in this particular phase is fear of separation. The discovery of the ego necessitates greater distance from the safe haven provided by the parents. But the child cannot yet survive on its own for very long. The core of its nature is still very sensitive and has the potential to be lastingly strengthened or distressed. This has an immediate effect on all four meridians of the second meridian family.

Instability within the family, a lack of care and attention or even rejection can lead the child to feel uncertain about his or her own position. As a result, the kidney meridian cannot fully develop since uncertainty is a poor substrate for discovering, exploring and expressing one's self and one's will. At the same time, the bladder meridian is overwhelmed due to the over-activation of the fight-or-flight mechanism. When you don't know for sure where you stand, you become cautious, even overly cautious; you're constantly in a state of tension. The small intestine meridian will therefore lose the strength to fulfil its separating function. It is afraid that it may find itself on its own. This hampers any further individuation. And the heart meridian begins to lack its zest for life since, overall, this is a situation that's not easy to bear. This may manifest as deep insecurity in the personality structure of the growing child and may turn into a life-determining topic in the adult. The deep longing for stability and validation can result in subordinating the core of our nature and its development to a continual examination of our deficits, rather than dealing with the core questions of the second meridian family.

No matter what happens during the developmental stage of the second meridian family, the first meridian family must always be considered as well. It is the base and forms the foundation. The seed of basic trust and confidence sown during the phase of the first meridian family sprouts during the time of the second meridian family. Stable basic trust provides a safe foundation so that it's much easier to cope with any unexpected earthquakes, such as parents divorcing. There will be considerably fewer cracks and dents in the wall of the soul. However, if the second meridian family sits on a weak foundation, it requires a lot of attention, affection and security to prevent it from crumbling away.

This has to do with the hierarchy of needs: only when existential needs are secure will there be time and space to deal with one's self and one's desires. It's a little bit like the balance in your bank account: if you have to watch every penny every single month to avoid your account being blocked, you'll hardly be contemplating questions about what you really want to achieve in your life. But an account with a healthy balance provides you with the freedom necessary to pursue precisely those questions. The first meridian family ensures that we are carried by the feeling that we're able to nourish and care for ourselves on all levels. And if it doesn't do that, it binds the energy of the second meridian family so that we're not following our will but our hunger. We don't live for our potential but for our bank account.

The second meridian family develops predominantly until about age six. The toddler matures to (pre)school age. During this period, many further aspects of the heart, small intestine, kidney and bladder meridians evolve – for example, imagination, thinking, a sense of time. The child will be able to refer to the past and have an image of the future. It will have a mental concept of itself. A further physical change will be imminent: the first teeth begin to fall out, the child-like facial features disappear, the bodily proportions change, arms and legs get longer relative to the torso, and the centre of gravity changes location. The next life phase begins; the third meridian family is knocking on the door, and along with it the adventure called the big wide world. What was sown during the time of the first meridian family and sprouted during the time of the second will now come to fruition.

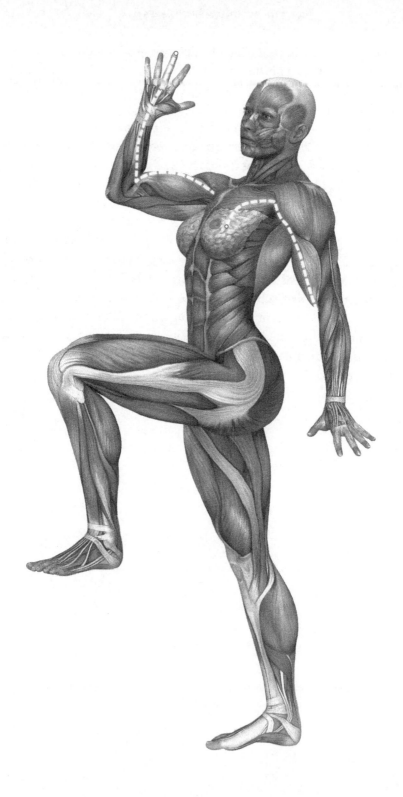

Chapter 13

The Pericardium Meridian

The Minister of Joy

Questions for the Pericardium Meridian

- Am I able to allow intimacy in the sense of familiarity and connectedness?
- Am I able to let people enter closely into my life?
- Am I able to allow closeness?
- Am I able to open up or close emotionally according to the circumstances and requirements?
- Am I highly sensitive? Am I easily touched or hurt?
- Am I able to enjoy myself? Am I able to enjoy pleasures and delights?
- Do I cultivate a large social network?
- Am I able to live and enjoy my sexuality satisfactorily?

The Life Principle of the Pericardium Meridian

In TCM, the pericardium meridian is considered the heart protector. The heart is the emperor of the organs, and the pericardium is his bodyguard. It decides who and what may or may not approach the emperor. The pericardium plays an important buffering role for the sensitive ruler. It is the first to deal with all welcome and unwelcome requests to the heart, and therefore it is also the heart's envoy. The pericardium conveys all the requests to the heart and, conversely, the heart's messages back to the external world. If the life principle of the pericardium is well developed, it endows us with the ability to open or close our hearts as required. We are able to consciously allow emotions and people to come near us or to reject them. We are able to manage our emotions.

This conscious opening and closing is important for pursuing a further core function: the pericardium is the minister of joy. In this context, joy may also refer to pleasure, especially pleasure regarding our interpersonal relationships. In order to experience and feel this pleasure, the emperor needs to leave his palace and engage in actual encounters. With the support and help of a strong pericardium meridian, he is perfectly able to do that. The pericardium meridian likes people, it enjoys talking to them and having an exchange with them. It likes hugging them and sleeping with them since, yes, sexuality is an important aspect of life and the pericardium meridian makes sure that it is taken care of sufficiently and satisfactorily.

In TCM, there is a close connection between the heart and the lower abdomen, with the pericardium meridian forming the bridge between the two. The pericardium connects lust and love; otherwise, things get either too physical or too emotional. Only with the right balance can the intimate exchange with another person become a holistic experience. Only then can the energy between two persons flow and circulate freely. The pericardium meridian is, after all, the master of circulation. The cardiovascular system, too, falls under its remit, so that sometimes the pericardium meridian is also referred to as the cardiovascular meridian. In this capacity, it once again serves as the heart's emissary. The heart's messages are represented by the blood, and it is the task of the pericardium meridian to distribute the blood in the entire body, from head to toe. Each cell is supplied with oxygen and nutrients. Blood and energy must circulate to even the most remote corners of our body-state. From there the blood returns laden with information. The pericardium meridian conveys, it relays and it integrates. A well-supplied and robust system feels well in itself. The pericardium meridian knows how to cultivate this feelgood factor, with sport and exercise playing an important role.

The pericardium meridian's task of circulation and integration also includes the psycho-emotional level. Its strength is social competence, building and maintaining networks, including friendships, acquaintances and romances. This is where it likes to circulate, where it knows how to integrate, perhaps even integrating those less integrated. It knows that networks also have a buffer function and are therefore able to protect the heart when it is unwell. Networks are the place where people can let their hair down and pour out their heart. It's where they find support and backing. It's where they are carried and cared for. But if the life principle of the pericardium meridian is only poorly developed, people will have problems dealing with emotional closeness. They will also find it difficult to open their hearts or protect their hearts – this includes the entire spectrum from having a heart of stone at one end to a heart of gold at the other. Some people don't like being touched. Or they don't like touching. Or they are touched too much. Or they touch too much. Or they oscillate between two extremes: open, closed, open, closed. Whichever it is, such people are emotionally vulnerable and find it hard to deal with all those aspects of life that characterise the pericardium meridian. This is not much fun. Accordingly, joy will find it hard to make an appearance.

For social beings like humans, the life principle of the pericardium meridian is an important factor for health and contentment. It concerns itself with matters of the heart, with closeness and with fun. When our pericardium meridian is well developed, we won't be lacking any of these.

The Pericardium Meridian and the Body

The Armoured Heart and Pressure

The word 'pericardium' comprises two words, 'around' and 'heart'. The pericardium is the heart sac, a connective tissue sac that surrounds the heart, providing it with freedom of movement by means of a thin lubricating layer, but also protecting the heart from over-expanding. This is precisely what the heart needs: protection as well as freedom of movement. In cases of an armoured heart (constrictive pericarditis), the pericardium thickens and becomes scarred, impairing the heart's ability to expand as the heart chambers are trying to fill up. During advanced stages, the heart sac becomes virtually rigid so that the heart is trapped as if wearing armour, and it becomes unable to fulfil its functions correctly. The hardening of the pericardium is caused by recurring inflammations, but what triggers them cannot always be determined.

TCM has recognised the idea of the armoured heart for more than 2000 years. But the definition of the space taken up by the heart has been extended to encompass the entire chest, the grand imperial palace, where the emperor should feel safe and move freely. The palace is safeguarded by the pericardium meridian: its pathway begins directly next to the heart and it controls exactly those muscles that are responsible for opening and closing the chest, in particular the major pectoral muscle. When this is tense, the chest will contract inwards and turn into armour: hard, limiting, rigid, inaccessible. The heart becomes withdrawn, locked into its own home, which gets ever more oppressive. The resulting tension impairs respiration and in turn leads to poorer circulation. This causes the body to constrict the blood vessels so that free movement and vitality are impaired in the entire area. It is no longer optimally supplied, perhaps even undersupplied, both physically and emotionally. In addition, the constriction leads to a build-up of pressure. The combination of pressure and constriction doesn't bode well for the heart. The heart protector has the task of keeping the emperor healthy. TCM therefore associates a disorder of the pericardium meridian not only with an armoured heart but also with many other cardiovascular diseases.

When the chest is hemmed in, the pericardium meridian will run into problems with its role as emissary. With everything locked down and tensed up, the energy and the blood need more pressure to get through. Here's a simple analogy, which is so often proven true in our everyday life. The tendency to high blood pressure can be well correlated with people who are under a lot of pressure, and whose life and wiggle room has become extremely tight while at the same time being under enormous strain – until their heart bursts. Hypertension rarely occurs in isolation; it has far-reaching consequences, especially affecting the blood vessels, whose interior walls can be affected by the constant high pressure. In damaged areas, there can be deposits of calcium, fat and connective tissue, which can further weaken or impair blood circulation. This is referred to as atherosclerosis. In the vocabulary of TCM, this is described as the emissary of the heart struggling to tour the empire. The roads are clogged up and in poor condition. An excursion to the farthest reaches of the body becomes increasingly difficult, even impossible. The consequences are circulatory disorders, in the hands, the legs, the head. It gets particularly nasty when the coronary vessels are affected. Typical signs of this happening are tightness sensations and pain in the chest as well as breathlessness (dyspnoea) with only little exertion. A small blood clot can lead to complete vascular obstruction; final destination: heart attack.

What can be done? Western medicine turns to brute measures using nitroglycerine, which, by the way, is a component of dynamite. Whether used internally or externally, explosives will clear clogged-up roads. If that doesn't help, long-term constricted areas get stretched surgically. In contrast, dealing with the life principle of the pericardium meridian is a much gentler approach. However, this should be started in good time, well before parts of the heart begin to die away, especially since the heart already starts to wither much earlier, not physically but mentally and emotionally. Many people feel chest pain, or a stinging pain or tightness, even though the heart is perfectly healthy. These are referred to as functional cardiac disorders. TCM would describe these as a disharmony of the pericardium meridian which is a bit overzealous in doing its job. Ultimately, the armoured chest is nothing but a protective shield to isolate the heart-emperor, to let nothing get to him, to not let him feel anything that he shouldn't or doesn't want to feel. Underneath it all is fear of emotional closeness. A good heart protector will not only ward off anything unwanted, but it will also try to lead the emperor out of his misery, or else the armour will turn into a prison where the mighty ruler will inevitably waste away. If we can no longer feel anything, we have become heart-less. The energy of the heart is dead.

One of the tasks of the pericardium meridian is therefore to break the self-imposed iron band around the chest again and again. But how? This is a case where the pericardium has to show courage in its role as emissary. It has to ask the emperor what he really wants. It has to ask the emperor what is good for him. What does the heart desire? What does it enjoy? What makes it feel light-hearted and easy-going? Those who don't listen to their heart will be feeling their heart. In this context, the pericardium meridian will get help from the small intestine meridian, which is also considered a protector of the heart: its task is to separate. Together they can liberate the heart. Get rid of everything that constricts the emperor – sorrows, relationships, job, fear. The heaviest load has to be taken off the emperor's mind – and heart – before it crushes him. That's the only way he'll be able to take a deep breath once again. And along with the breath, blood, expansiveness and vitality will return to the chest. Instead of strangling its own heart, the pericardium meridian will be able to provide spaciousness and freedom once again. This will keep the heart healthy and protect it from hardening.

SYMPTOMS ASSOCIATED WITH THE PERICARDIUM MERIDIAN

A feeling of tension or tightness in the chest, difficulty breathing even after only light exertion, arrhythmia, claustrophobia, hypertension, coronary heart disease, myocardial infarction, functional heart disorders...

Running in Circles

In TCM, the pericardium meridian is one of the most essential controllers of the cardiovascular system and is therefore also referred to as the cardiovascular meridian. It facilitates blood circulation. As the emissary of the heart, it ensures that the entire empire is catered for. To this end, it requires pressure and strength, especially for reaching those frontiers which are at the furthest distance from the headquarters. When the pericardium meridian is weakened, its actions will be listless. It will no longer perambulate cheerfully and vigorously in order to disseminate the happy news contained in the blood; rather, it will hang about exhaustedly, with far-reaching consequences: the periphery will remain undersupplied, and blood pressure will be stuck in the basement.

This state of affairs is particularly evident in the hands, which, in TCM, have a direct relationship with the heart. Forget about a warm and welcoming handshake! Instead, cold, limp and slightly damp hands cautiously stretch out for a greeting. They lack energy, vitality, warmth. They lack cordiality. With such a handshake, you feel as if you're not really holding anything in your hands. You are afraid to give the hand a good shake as it seems to express deficiency and insecurity. The emperor does not show himself; he's hiding. This also manifests in the face, which is also seen as a mirror of the heart.

When there is a weakness in the pericardium meridian, the heart lacks the pressure required to bring sufficient blood to the head. The tendency to vertigo is coupled with a tendency to a noble pallor. There's a whiff of aristocracy, of a lofty distance from life, which is another aspect of how the pericardium meridian may present itself. Reserved and withdrawn in its palace, it observes from the balcony the pulsating life of the people with slight amazement or wonderment but without wanting or being able to participate. That's because the legs are, of course, also weak and malnourished. You won't get far with them, and certainly not fast, without running the risk of collapse or fainting. You are devoid of any power and therefore prefer to be in a horizontal position where the blood can be distributed in the body on its own account. The emperor lies exhaustedly on the floor. He is too tired to face life. People notice this condition particularly in the morning: getting up turns into a form of torture and should only be performed in slow motion; otherwise, they may simply collapse. Men are hit by this condition doubly hard: impotent wimps, both psychologically and physically. A weakened pericardium meridian can result in a weak cardiovascular system and low blood pressure. In such cases, the heart protector protects the heart by using its symptoms to keep the emperor away from life to avoid overburdening him. But how to nurse him back to health?

The heart protector has to take his life more into his own hands, he has to reclaim his capacity for action, he has to handle life differently, he has to move. However, TCM derides sport as practised in our Western culture – and for a good reason: we often take it much too seriously. There's always a sense of having to perform, to become faster, stronger, healthier. It gets really absurd when people who are already stressed after a demanding twelve-hour day go and train for a marathon or try to bust the gym with heavy weights. Such an approach to exercise stands a good chance of exacerbating any stress and overwhelm, to the point that the heart may break, despite all the healthy training.

The most important function of exercise is to gently give the emperor a leg up and strengthen him. Exercising should stimulate the circulation in his body and build up, rather than use up, his energy. The form of health cultivation established in Asia, therefore, mainly comprises gentle forms of movement, which address not only the body but also the mind. These types of exercise are ideal for people with low blood pressure and a poor cardiovascular system. They meet the emperor where they find him: a bit down.

SYMPTOMS ASSOCIATED WITH THE PERICARDIUM MERIDIAN

Low blood pressure, unstable blood pressure, vertigo, circulatory disorders, difficulty concentrating, getting tired easily, increased desire for sleep, lack of drive, depressive mood, spontaneous sweating...

The Pericardium Meridian and the Psyche

The Heart Protector

Approximately 15–20% of the population are considered highly sensitive and are actually referred to as highly sensitive persons (HSPs). Put differently, one could also say that about 15–20% of the population do not have a pericardium meridian with a fully developed life principle. The pericardium meridian protects the heart. If it doesn't fulfil its task sufficiently, all kinds of stimuli reach the heart directly and unfiltered. Such people are easily affected by just about anything and take everything to heart. They are emotionally highly strung, easily upset and ruffled; they are quickly distracted, overwrought, distressed, hurt. In other words, they are highly sensitive persons.

Sensitivity per se is a beautiful quality as it represents a finely tuned discernment for people and situations, an excellent eye for details and nuances, an almost magical intuition, great empathy and lateral thinking. But walking around today's performance-oriented culture with a constantly open and soft heart is not always comfortable, either for the person concerned or for their environment, which more often than not will lack any understanding of such a hypersensitive state. A well-developed pericardium meridian can be of great help in this scenario: it puts itself between the heart and any input. It acts like a buffer or an airbag; it gives the emperor time to prepare himself for the constantly arising external impressions so that he's not confronted by them directly and unexpectedly. The pericardium meridian facilitates a conscious closing of the heart, a conscious withdrawal, a sensible distancing from emotional turbulences so that the emperor can stay grounded. It dampens the sensory overload to a tolerable extent.

This is very important because a heart that is too open is like an invitation: Everybody welcome! Just come in and trample on my feelings to your heart's delight! Without a protective pericardium meridian, you might be easily influenced by the moods of the people around you since it's difficult for you to differentiate between the internal and external world. You feel what the other person feels. You experience what the other person experiences. You mirror what's going on in the other person. You adapt in an attempt to acquiesce. You really don't want to provoke a conflict. Because any disharmony is like a direct hit at your heart, and that is, of course, something that you'd like to avoid. Without protective armour, people quickly react to pressure and stress. There is constant overstimulation, a continual state of hyperarousal, permanent tension. This is inhibiting as you tend to be overwhelmed, either by the situation itself or by perceived expectations. For this reason, a weakness of the pericardium meridian often goes hand in hand with timidity, reclusiveness and fearfulness, or even social phobias.

The converse situation isn't easy either. A pericardium meridian that takes its task too seriously turns people into a bull in a china shop. They roll like an indestructible tank through life, leaving numerous piles of shards in their wake, which they are completely unaware of. What they lack is empathy, for other people and also for themselves. Often there will be a valid reason for this; perhaps at some point in their development it was necessary to squeeze into a protective armour that would make everything bounce off. But if the causative necessity is in the past and they are still in their armour in the present, these people's reaction to life will be hard, rigid, inflexible, especially regarding emotional issues. One could describe them as HIPs, highly insensitive persons – or emotionally stunted persons. Such people won't let anything get close to them since closeness can be dangerous. And if it looks as though closeness may be in the offing, then they will stop it in its tracks as a precautionary measure. Their defence mechanism can be strong enough to destroy love. They are good at dishing out but not good at being on the receiving end, especially where matters of the heart are concerned. There is no more enticing, just blocking. Perhaps it's for a reason that the pericardium meridian ends at the middle finger: back off! The heart expresses itself with a gesture of the deepest contempt.

The pericardium meridian is the gate to the heart. And this gate can be too open or too firmly closed. Sometimes a disharmony of the pericardium meridian can lead to a constant oscillating between these two extremes, between exaggerated reticence and exaggerated approachability. One moment, a person is fully present and could hug the entire world and love everything and everyone; the next, they've suddenly gone to ground in their shell, unreachable by anyone at all. One moment, a full emotional discharge; the next, utter avoidance of any emotions at all. They are unable to consciously control this shuttling, they are entirely at its mercy. And yet it's precisely the capacity for consciously controlling the gate that distinguishes the life principle of the pericardium meridian. A healthy pericardium meridian is a responsible gatekeeper, a wise protector of the heart. It knows precisely what it allows through to the emperor and at what time, and also what it has to keep out and when. This knowledge leads to a high degree of sovereignty and self-determination in emotional matters.

Let's Talk About Sex

Sex needs the body. Love needs the soul. In order to unite these two aspects, you need the pericardium meridian. Otherwise, sex and love would be two separate and independent areas of our lives, and there would be the danger of constantly feeling that something is missing. Where there is love, eroticism struggles, and sex is lacking closeness and feeling. However, a fulfilling sexuality, whether as a single person or within a relationship, is important for health and wellbeing – unless someone has decided to dedicate their lives exclusively to one goddess or one god or another spiritual path. And even if someone chooses this path, the transformation of sexual energy into pure love and pure light doesn't always work out. But if you are oriented towards a more worldly life, it's worthwhile listening to your pericardium meridian because being frustrated about your love life can have a direct effect on your heart. The pericardium meridian, as the protector of the emperor of all organs, strives to avoid such frustration by promoting a holistic approach in people's relationships based on its competence in matters of circulation, integration and opening the heart.

A well-developed pericardium meridian allows us to experience deep and true intimacy. A hallmark of intimacy is our ability to experience touch, connectedness and familiarity not only on a physical but also on an emotional and mental level. Without this kind of intimacy, sex is simply about the meeting of two egocentric people seeking their own satisfaction and trying to achieve this in a purely physical way. That's not always a bad thing. Sometimes sex simply has the purpose of a cleansing catharsis: pressure, tension, lust, desire, drive – all this needs a valve; it wants to be lived and burned, ideally in the fire of passion, right now in the present moment. It's easy to get intimate in this way; it can happen very quickly, within a few hours or minutes, if that's how it has to be. It corresponds to the current zeitgeist to feel the need for satisfying cravings without any delay. However, if serendipity doesn't bring the love of your life but a similarly libidinous person instead, breakfast may well be in the form of the 'lovely night but it's the morning after' syndrome. No matter how many coalescing orgasms there may have been, no matter how ecstatic the sensual frenzy, there will be a strange feeling of emptiness, of not being sure what to do with the person lying next to you in bed, feeling out of place. That's quite simply because something is missing. Something that cannot be dealt with by a one-night stand.

The heart begins to blossom when it is cared for by the trinity of love. It needs intimacy in the form of emotional closeness and familiarity, it needs passion in the form of romantic and passionate lust, and it needs connectedness, loyalty and stability. Love without passion and connectedness is purely sex. The pericardium meridian has the capacity to bring together and connect all these qualities. It facilitates the conscious change between different levels. Sometimes we need more of a particular level, sometimes our partner needs more of another one. The pericardium meridian allows us to choose, to play, to decide. It is clear for the pericardium what it's all about.

This is important since otherwise we would be looking on the wrong level for what's missing – generally, the physical level, because it is the most accessible. This can lead to feelings of needing more and yet more, without ever getting enough. It can even lead to being addicted to sex, which is considered a malfunction of the pericardium meridian. For others, the opposite is the case: for them, the path to the nether regions is via the heart and the heart alone. This, too, is a disharmony of the pericardium meridian. It is impossible to feel lust unless closeness and connectedness are a factor. Sexual intercourse turns into an exercise in confirming love. You make love in order to be loved. You can only make love when you are loved. A little vicious circle, which tends to result in an uptight way of dealing with the whole sex thing. Lust can thus lose its animalistic aspect and libidinous vitality, instead turning ever more into a lack of lust, until, finally, you've reached a dead end. This is also a form of imbalance which can gnaw away at a contented atmosphere in the bedroom.

When it is in a healthy and vibrant state, the pericardium meridian supports the balance between physical, emotional and mental factors. It opens the heart, but also the pelvis, providing it with blood and energy. It allows our lust to circulate in our entire body. It is the key to a truly satisfying sexuality.

Signs of an Imbalanced and Balanced Pericardium Meridian

Signs of an Imbalanced Pericardium Meridian

- Hypersensitivity, emotionally very vulnerable
- Emotional coldness, emotionally stunted, withdrawn, distant

- Emotionally 'hot and cold', oscillating between being reserved and approachable, between emotional discharge and avoidance
- Problems with closeness, intimacy and fulfilling sexuality
- Circulatory disorders, tendency to high or low blood pressure, susceptible to heart disorders
- Difficulty with pleasure and fun, or addicted to pleasure and sex

Signs of a Balanced Pericardium Meridian

- Conscious control regarding emotions, conscious opening and closing
- No fear of intimacy, familiarity, connectedness
- Sexually fulfilled on all levels, enjoying intimacy
- High social competence, much empathy
- Robust cardiovascular system, stable blood pressure, good circulation

How to Strengthen the Life Principle of the Pericardium Meridian

Hugging

Hugging is the most important exercise for the pericardium meridian! A good hug is both easy and difficult, as it involves so much more than just putting your arms round someone. Make it your goal to hug one person a day. You don't have anybody at home? Then catch someone at work. There's always a reason or an opportunity to give someone a hug. But you need to be mindful that you don't just hug physically. Hug with your heart! Before you spread your arms, briefly gather your focus in your chest, trying to feel the lower tip of your heart. Then begin the movement from there, with your external movement following your internal movement; open up yourself and all your senses. And then take the other person into your heart. Try to continue to feel the tip of your heart and enter into a connection with the other person. Try to relax deeply and to soften your body. Breathe deeply and freely. Stay like this for ten seconds at least. You will be surprised!

The Rose Hedge

Imagine a beautiful rose hedge growing all around you. You're standing in the centre, with the hedge surrounding you in a circle. Now configure the hedge according to your taste: its height, density, the colour of the flowers, the size of the thorns. Do this visualisation several times a day. At first when you have a quiet moment, then in public spaces, in the underground, on the bus, on the pavement. Then do it while you're interacting with other people. The hedge is your protective shield. No one can penetrate it. Words and feelings are filtered by the hedge. Anything that could harm you or could get too close to you gets caught by the thorns or is absorbed by the flowers. Within the shelter of the hedge, all you perceive is the beautiful scent of the roses. Try to visualise this image so strongly that you can remain relaxed and open within your rose hedge, even if someone is trying to harass you emotionally.

The Pathway of the Pericardium Meridian

The pericardium meridian arises in the fourth intercostal space at Pericardium 1, one thumb-width lateral to the nipple. From there, it ascends in a straight line towards the shoulder, to just above the armpit. It then follows the border of the great chest muscle (pectoralis major) to the upper arm where the pericardium meridian runs between the two heads of the biceps brachii to reach its clearly palpable tendon in the elbow crease. Pericardium 3 is located in the centre of the elbow crease, on the little-finger side of the biceps tendon.

The meridian continues along the midline of the forearm, initially coursing slightly more medially – that is, closer to the little finger. After about a third of the way, it veers to travel exactly in the middle, between the two pronounced muscles and tendons of the flexor carpi radialis and the palmaris longus. Pericardium 6 is located between these two tendons, two thumb-widths proximal to the wrist crease. The centre of the wrist crease, again between those same tendons, is the location of Pericardium 7, while the centre of the palm, between the third and fourth metacarpal bones, is the site of Pericardium 8. From the centre of the inside of the hand, the pericardium meridian continues towards the middle finger, where it runs along its inner midline to its tip, where it terminates with Pericardium 9 at the highest point of the finger.

Key Areas of the Pericardium Meridian

Chest

The chest is the palace of the heart: here resides the emperor. And it's also the location of the alarm point of the heart, Ren Mai 14, *ju que* or 'Great Palace', situated two thumb-widths below the tip of the sternum. The emperor's alarm bells ring when his palace gets too cramped or doesn't provide sufficient protection. That's the task of the pericardium meridian, whose alarm point is in the exact centre of the sternum: Ren Mai 17, *shan zhong* or 'Chest Centre'. This point is also the meeting point of any form of energy, emphasising the importance of the heart for the entire body. An imbalance in the pericardium meridian can therefore affect the vitality of the whole chest and manifests in these two key points.

The pericardium meridian begins one thumb-width lateral to the nipple at the point Pericardium 1, *tian chi* or 'Heavenly Pool'. The meridian connects the pectoralis and the biceps. The transitional area between the two muscles is the location of the point Pericardium 2, *tian quan* or 'Heavenly Spring'. When tensed, the muscle chain formed by the pectoralis major and the biceps closes the chest. The shoulders are pulled forward and inward, and the arms to the body, while the centre of the breastbone pulls back. Continuous tension in this area can lead to the build-up of a veritable armour. People withdraw into their shell. The connection to heaven and the expansiveness of life is severed. Red alert for the emperor who gets under pressure and feels suffocated by the tight chest.

When this muscle chain is only poorly developed, the result is a weak chest. Little tone, little protection. Once again, the emperor's alarm bells will be ringing. He will be prone to a nervous disposition since he is more or less naked – no armour, no gatekeeper. In an ideal world, the powerful heart with its proud chest has the capacity to present itself with openness and vitality.

Forearm and Hand

The pericardium meridian controls the forearm musculature required to form a fist. This corresponds to the pericardium's function of heart protector. We may welcome someone with open hands – or we may threaten them with our fist or show someone our middle finger. We can keep the door to our heart open or closed. This is expressed by the point Pericardium 6, *nei guan* or 'Inner Gate', which is located on the middle of the forearm, two thumb-widths above the wrist crease. Closing Pericardium 6 is like making a fist, and the door to our heart closes; we are prepared to defend ourselves, which we also signal with the point Pericardium 9, *zhong chong* or 'Central Surge', located in the centre of the tip of the middle finger. The fist clenched, the middle finger stretched out, the canons are charged. Get lost, all of you. The onslaught has been warded off.

This certainly can't be a permanent solution. If we are constantly busy fighting off any perceived attacks, sooner or later this will seriously concern the emperor since such a state isn't in accordance with his true nature. In the centre of the palm is the point Pericardium 8, *lao gong* or 'Palace of Weariness'; a palace that turns into a prison is a place of weariness. It is therefore crucial to open the clenched fist and to return to life by extending one's hand.

The Pericardium Meridian: Key Points

- Associated element: Fire element
- Quality: Yin
- Time on the organ clock: 7pm–9pm
- Animal quality: Dog
- Partner meridian: Triple heater meridian
- Twinned meridian: Liver meridian
- Opposite meridian: Stomach meridian

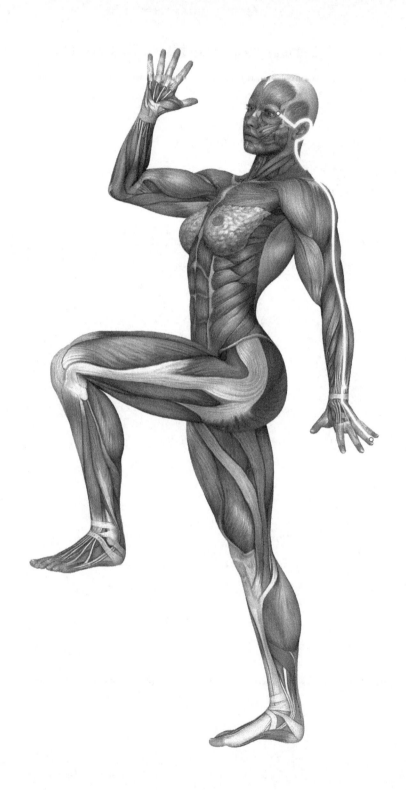

Chapter 14

The Triple Heater Meridian

Coordination and Homoeostasis

Questions for the Triple Heater Meridian

- Do I have a sense of my inner balance? Am I able to create this for myself?
- Am I able to coordinate all the areas of my life that are important to me?
- Am I able to self-regulate and control myself?
- Am I able to adapt and integrate well?
- Do I have a robust physical, mental and emotional resilience?
- Am I able to remain stable and centred during times of change?
- Am I able to process and resolve emotional hurt within an appropriate time frame?
- Do I often feel ambivalent?
- Do I easily feel conflicted inside?
- Do I have a healthy and robust metabolism?

The Life Principle of the Triple Heater Meridian

Of the twelve main meridians, the triple heater is the only one without a direct relationship to a particular organ. In TCM, it is said that the triple heater has a function without form. In fact, it doesn't need a form since it is our body's most important overall coordinator. It has to be on top of things; it has to be above it all, with a little bit of distance. It will lend a hand where it is needed. And it is needed all the time since building a team with eleven meridians that need to pull together, each with its distinctive leanings and talents, is not easy. The triple heater's most important role is controlling metabolism: all organs, all regulatory mechanisms, all cycles have to be finely tuned and interact harmoniously. The triple heater meridian therefore provides a healthy steady state for well-functioning homoeostasis, a task comprising both the emotional as well as the physical realm. It helps us to maintain a well-balanced inner state; it facilitates stability, consistency and integration.

In this way, the triple heater meridian endows us with the ability to successfully reconcile all important aspects of our lives. The classic work–life balance is one of its easier tasks; a triple heater with a well-developed life principle ensures a balanced ratio between work and leisure. However, the triple heater is not concerned about meaningfully dividing hours and seconds among the different needs; rather, it works continuously on the ultimate masterplan, with the aim of integrating all its various aspects into one big entity. It is like a seismograph registering the smallest tremor in the foundations of our individual harmony. If there are discrepancies between what is and what is desired, the triple heater can correct these since, in its role as coordinator, it is mindful of the greater picture and has a firm hand on the tiller. Or not.

If there is a weakness in the triple heater meridian, this balancing principle will be missing. Fire on the roof, water in the basement. Whether it's affecting our external life or our metabolism, some areas will escalate completely, while others will be dismally starving. A derailment, a separation, a destabilisation. The head has nothing to do with the body, nor the family with leisure time, breadwinning with meaning in life, respiration with the belly, or the kidneys with the heart. Each area wants to have its own way; there is no communal plan, no communal goal. This leads to conflicts of interest, inner tension, discord, incompatibility, disorientation. The bottom line is turmoil, fragmentation, a gross imbalance, with the ensuing friction consuming vast amounts of energy. This weakens the body, both emotionally and physically. It predisposes us to all kinds of disturbing influences, even though protecting us from such influences is precisely what should be an integral part of the triple heater's life principle.

TCM considers the triple heater a protective shield, which, together with the lungs, defends us against external influences. The triple heater represents our immunity, our resilience, psychologically and emotionally. When the triple heater energy is strong, we are forearmed against cold, heat, wind or dampness, against conflicts, emotional injuries, shock or trauma... We're able to deal with and process boundary violations. The triple heater protects and guards, through either defence or adaptation. It can be strong, but it can also bend like bamboo, without losing its balance or identity, or straying from its destiny. The triple heater stands for our body's bamboo principle. It adjusts to the wind without breaking.

Based on its ability to adapt, the triple heater meridian is sometimes referred to as the travel meridian since travelling generally means accommodating new stimuli and new situations. During a holiday, a weak triple heater may easily panic when the beer tastes different from that at home, when the bed is too soft or too hard or too short or too narrow. No adaptability: people try to maintain a rigid balance at any price, and in doing so lose it even more. They find it hard to surrender to an unfamiliar dynamic or to adjust to new challenges. But this refers not only to journeys to far-flung regions but also to the most important journey of all – the journey of our life. Without a well-functioning triple heater, people quickly begin to stagnate or tread water when processes requiring change invite them to leave their comfort zone. Because they are afraid of reorganising their lives. This is a far cry from the state indicative of a healthy triple heater meridian: a unity of body, mind and spirit, and a life in which all aspects are finely tuned and interact harmoniously, providing a vibrant tailwind.

The Triple Heater Meridian and the Body

Providing and Metabolising Form

In TCM, the torso is divided into three areas, with each area allocated a particular task. The chest governs circulation and distribution. The upper abdomen controls digestion, while the lower abdomen is responsible for elimination. The logistics centre is above, production is in the middle, drainage below. Three areas, three chambers, three tasks. As is the case in all areas of our life, fulfilling these tasks optimally requires energy and warmth, and it's for this reason that TCM talks about the three burners or heaters. The fire of life has to circulate in all three heaters to keep the entire organism healthy and vibrant.

The triple heater connects the three chambers to form one huge functional unit which could be described as our metabolism – the foundation for all vital processes in our body. Each cell requires sufficient supplies, each cell has to dispose of any waste, all matter has to be exchanged continuously, and all regulatory mechanisms should be fine-tuned accordingly. There is, of course, not just the one metabolism. Carbohydrates, protein, fats and minerals all need to be metabolised, and in addition there needs to be anabolism and catabolism. The bottom line: there is a lot the triple heater meridian has to deal with. And such a complex job profile is consequently quite susceptible to disturbances.

Homoeostasis refers to the body's or a system's ability to maintain a balanced and steady internal state. A strong triple heater energy is perfectly capable of achieving just that. It provides a dynamic metabolic harmony. Conversely, any imbalances of the triple heater can have far-reaching effects. When the fire in the chambers subsides, the heaters become congested as they can no longer fulfil their respective tasks adequately. When the circulation is blocked in the upper heater, the breathing becomes very shallow, and the head is hemmed in by a helmet of fog and lethargy. When the digestion is blocked in the middle heater, the digestive fire doesn't burn properly, and the food is converted only inadequately. People like that put on weight simply by contemplating eating a piece of cake. And blocked elimination in the lower heater will affect the stools or urine or both. All this dampens down energy levels, mood, mental focus, immunity. Mountains of garbage pile up because elimination takes place only half-heartedly, and people may suffer from oedema or gout. The metabolism is in the doldrums. It is in urgent need of a boost; it needs some fire under its corpulent backside. It needs a strong triple heater meridian.

Conversely, the triple heater can also be a bit too motivated, trying to light the candle with a flamethrower, so to speak. Then it will burn down everything that gets in its way. Matter is metabolised faster than it can be eliminated. The only positive effect is that people like that can eat as much as they want and still lose weight. And the price they pay for this? Nervousness, palpitations, trembling, sweating, hypertension, insomnia. The thyroid is buzzing and overactive. Our resources are being nibbled on. When the triple heater becomes derailed, so too does the control of the fire: it can blaze and burn us. Or it can just smoulder, and we miss its effects. The resting metabolic rate can be too high or too low. Or someone may oscillate between two extremes. Sometimes like this, sometimes like that. It can be too hot or chilled like ice, full of energy or completely knackered. The energy balance is like a roller coaster. This, too, can be an expression of an imbalance in the triple heater meridian.

You could imagine the triple heater meridian as a thermostat. When it functions well, it automatically adjusts the temperature to the prevailing conditions and provides an ideal ambient temperature so that everybody feels comfortable. But if it is out of control, it may be heating up the room even if it's 30 degrees outside. Or it doesn't heat, even though there are several feet of snow outside. Or it heats at night but not during the day. Or it heats in a rhythm that doesn't make sense. The house suffers. Sometimes mould builds up on the walls; at other times, everything dries out. It's impossible to feel truly at home in such a house. The physiological imbalance clouds the psychological balance. It covers the whole range from apathy to irritation or oscillates between the two. Everything is possible, except emotional or mental stability. But when the triple heater is well developed, there is no better place than our body: everything runs smoothly, everything self-regulates; no extremes can throw us off course. We exude vibrant health.

Fatigue, lack of appetite, weight gain or weight loss, oedema, gout, urinary difficulties, metabolic syndrome, diabetes mellitus, irritable bowel syndrome, hyper/hypothyroidism...

Protective Shield and Integration

The point Triple Heater 5, *wai guan* or 'Outer Pass', is one of the most important points on the triple heater meridian. The triple heater meridian is like an outer pass or gate that protects us from influences that shouldn't penetrate our bodies. In TCM, the triple heater, together with the lung meridian, governs our defensive energy, which can be imagined like a protective shield. When this shield is strong, everything that could be harmful to us bounces off. If it is weak, it's like a welcome sign for any type of bad weather, both literally and emotionally. There is, however, one factor the triple heater reacts to especially sensitively, and that's wind. Wind is the climatic factor related to change and is therefore a particular challenge to the balance-loving triple heater.

For a triple heater with a poorly developed life principle, even the slightest breeze is enough to cause a stiff neck. You open the car window for just one minute, and the next day you're barely able to move. If you want to sleep with an open window, expect a bout of sciatica the next morning if the night breathed not just darkness but also cold and draughts into your bed. Wind is about change, and change requires adaptation, maintaining balance – or we will be blown over. Our capacity to deal with wind shows the strengths or weaknesses of the triple heater meridian. The same is true for the wind of life, which can also be quite rough at times.

This refers in particular to emotional attacks or infringements that often require a particularly strong protective shield. The triple heater is perfectly able to provide this and deflect boundary violations or assaults on our emotions. And even if a hurricane sweeps over the soulscape, tearing down fences, blowing off roofs – in other words, when there is shock, trauma or abuse – a strong triple heater will endow us with the capacity to repair any damage and rebuild the shaken-up inner balance. Of course, it can't fix or cope with everything. Some things simply can't be rebuilt, at least not in the way they were before. But the triple heater is the authority that has a strong say in how long and how intensely external factors that have forcefully entered our body will remain and how we deal with them.

A weakness of the triple heater meridian can have us grappling our entire life with the fact we didn't manage to blow out all the candles at our fourth birthday party or that we were picked up late from nursery one day. To be begin with, we craft a drama out of this, then we turn the drama into trauma, then we can't get rid of the trauma any more, and finally we develop pyrophobia, or shortness of breath when stressed, or fear of loss when someone is late. In adulthood, poor triple heater energy can be the reason we still haven't processed an argument with our partner a year later, or are still upset about losing a job ten years ago. The triple heater meridian is excellent at bearing a grudge. This is similar to how, on a physical level, a weak triple heater meridian has to fight for weeks to get over the slightest of colds, without ever really managing a breakthrough. Conversely, a strong triple heater meridian can handle even a severe shock affecting its balance with strength and confidence. It may get bent, but it won't break. It is able to integrate any kind of injuries and disturbances. Its nature is integrative.

As coordinator of the body's metabolism, and therefore of all organs and all functional and controlling circuits, the triple heater can't afford to neglect anything or anybody. It has to constantly pay attention to make sure that a cohesive, cooperating unit is formed and sustained. It gets everybody round the table. It connects. And it connects especially what we like to separate, such as our head and our body, thinking and feeling. This separation often occurs in the aftermath of traumatic events to prevent us from feeling what happened to us. For a certain period of time, such a protective mechanism makes perfect sense.

In the long run, however, a much more balanced self-image will arise by bringing all the unintegrated issues to the surface and making them a part of ourselves. And it can help to take a proper look at our blind spots which, having shut themselves off from the rest of the body, lead an independent existence that can disturb our entire organism. This is a scenario where the triple heater comes into its own: it will tidy up and make peace. It strives for all-encompassing harmony – the best protection possible. Because harmony results in more energy, vitality as well as physical and psycho-emotional immunity.

Weakened immunity, sensitivity to external influences (especially wind, but also against emotional injuries, noise, etc.), susceptible to changes in the weather, temperature sensitivity, stiff neck, stiff shoulders...

The Triple Heater Meridian and the Psyche

Adapting Needs a Good Fit

A lot can happen as you're sailing along in your boat on the ocean of life. Some people just drift or go round in a circle. Others know precisely which direction they want to take. Only a few have a clearly defined goal, and even if they do, it's all too easy to get off course. There may be unforeseen currents, the wind may change, storms may necessitate turning around. There isn't always a direct route from A to B. Those who can adapt have an easier time. And if you don't believe this, try sailing into the wind. It will only throw you back. Sometimes it requires skill to progress in the right direction: tack left, tack right, again and again. Sometimes we need to take detours. Sometimes we need to be flexible. The triple heater meridian endows us with the capacity to adapt to a change in circumstances or new challenges quickly and effortlessly, as well as keeping our ultimate goal in sight. It allows us to adapt without losing or giving up on ourselves. The triple heater considers flexibility as a broadening of our scope so that we can access meaningful alternatives for our progress while maintaining our principles and tenacity.

Weak triple heater energy can manifest itself in two ways. There can be either obstinacy or its opposite, so that even the most minute changes turn people into a weather vane. They accept whatever is going on; they make themselves small to avoid causing ripples. They make themselves invisible, allowing themselves to be formed, bent and broken. But this won't maintain their inner balance. It's thrown away instead. This is obsequiousness to the point of self-denial. External demands and expectations, rather than their own needs, values or desires, become their landmarks. These are conformists, yea-sayers, hypocrites, moral cowards. The triple heater's protective function has failed completely.

Exaggerated obstinacy represents the flip side of the coin and is equally non-constructive. If you stand stiffly in the middle of a hurricane, it's only a matter of time before you break or become uprooted. That's because it takes an extraordinary amount of energy and in the long run simply wears you down. The problem is that people often don't even recognise this happening. Furthermore, because of their limited scope of action, they lose the connection to their environment. They become disconnected. They're not really aware of what is going on around them and their response is there-fore maladapted. They constantly have the underlying feeling of being a round peg in a square hole or of being sidelined. Once again, the triple heater as the travel meridian provides a good explanation. When the triple heater doesn't do its job well, you could be living in a foreign country for 30 years without recognising the need to learn its language, to consider its cultural traits or to feel connected with its population. You can be in a job for 30 years without identifying with it in the slightest. You can be married to someone for 30 years without really having committed to your spouse.

It's for a reason that the wedding band is worn on precisely the finger that is part of the pathway of the triple heater meridian. When living closely together, what could be more important than adaptability without loss of identity? It allows the maintaining of healthy homoeostasis between two individuals. The triple heater meridian gives us the ability to quickly fine-tune our behaviour according to the requirements of the most diverse situations. It allows us to change and realign our behavioural patterns if this would serve some supraordinate goal. It stands for adaptable and fluid structures in our relationships. In this context, the triple heater directs all other meridians. It reins in where reining in is necessary; it promotes and demands as required, always with an eye on the path and the goal.

Self-Regulation and Self-Control

The life principle of the triple heater is homoeostasis. Homoeostasis refers to the ability to maintain a certain inner balance while adjusting to changing life conditions. This includes self-responsibly balancing psychological tension since balanced emotional and mental states contribute considerably to our wellbeing and overall health. But this balance is quite fragile given that it's frequently put to the test and challenged by the dynamics and demands of our lives. We all find ourselves constantly exposed to charged opinions, expectations, needs, emotions and values. We live and experience our life with all its heights and all its depths. We are happy, sad, content, angry.

It goes with the territory that we lose our balance for short periods of time – and regain it. For the latter to happen, we need the triple heater. Its task is not only maintaining but also re-establishing homoeostasis on all levels. A triple heater with a well-developed life principle can quickly smooth out any emotional or mental turmoil. The bamboo principle allows the wind to shake us, but afterwards we promptly straighten up again. A robust triple heater will take the thunderstorm of an argument in its stride. Life's too short, life goes on. But people with a weak triple heater will get stuck in emotional loops. They buckle and take a long time to stand up straight again. However, sometimes there can be storms or headwinds that really throw us off course. Then the triple heater meridian has to interfere. It provides us with the capacity of conscious self-regulation. It helps us to control, process and influence our thoughts and feelings.

In its role as coordinator, the triple heater meridian is able to stay on top of things and be cognisant of the overall situation. It allows us to consider our behaviour in a reflective yet distanced manner. This is important in order to recognise the discrepancy between how things are and how we would like them to be. A desired condition does not represent a fixed state but can be changed according to the current stage of our life, our goals and needs. For example, we desire a harmonious relationship with our partner. Day after day, however, our choleric boss succeeds in poisoning our mind, which we have struggled to balance during our morning meditation. By the end of the day, all we manage is to trudge home in a grumpy mood. And once at home, we offload our frustration on precisely the person we have been looking forward to seeing all day. A strong triple heater energy is able to intervene in such a situation. It weighs up what is important and right for us against what is expected, required or demanded from us, economically, socially or simply in practical terms. And the triple heater corrects. When it notices that our inner balance is so much out of kilter that there is a stagnant or destructive milieu, it has the necessary competence to step in.

If the worst comes to the worst, it's better to hand in your notice and look for another job. Or take measures in the workplace, speak to your boss, establish better boundaries. Or let off steam before going home, have a quick session at the gym or scream your head off in the car; rage, shout, swear – whatever it takes to re-establish your inner ecology so that you can meet your partner with an open heart. The life principle of the triple heater allows us to consciously self-regulate and manage ourselves. It knows which screws it has to turn so that the artistic synthesis of our life script can run smoothly. It makes us exercise when we have put on too many pounds; it makes us cultivate our friendships when we feel lonely; it makes us transform anger that is eating up our insides.

When there is a weakness in the life principle of the triple heater meridian, we lack the distance and overview for self-reflection. We get bogged down when faced with a problem. We find ourselves in a cul-de-sac but are unable to simply turn round and walk the other way. We are unable to activate ourselves, we lack the competence to work towards a solution. Defeat, calamities and losses are all very difficult to cope with. You tend to respond impulsively and situationally. You're not able to control yourself or your emotions since poor self-regulation comes with poor self-control. You react rather than act. And those who can't regulate themselves tend to be unable to regulate their lives either.

The triple heater meridian allows us to stand up and continue time and again. In times of crisis, it helps us to remain calm and act with careful consideration. It helps us to stay on course and regain our inner balance and stability through goal-oriented actions in accordance with reality.

Signs of an Imbalanced and Balanced Triple Heater Meridian

Signs of an Imbalanced Triple Heater Meridian

— Easily getting unbalanced

— Easily losing control of self and emotions

— Compartmentalisation of different aspects of life

— Frequent inner conflicts and strife

— Lack of unity of body and mind

— Difficulties in adapting to new challenges

— Sensitivity towards external influences, such as wind or emotional attacks or violations

— Tendency to metabolic disorders

Signs of a Balanced Triple Heater Meridian

— Capacity for self-regulation and self-control

— High adaptability when faced with challenges or change

— Inner balance and stability

— Body and mind balanced and in harmony

— Good integration and coordination of all areas of life

— Good defence mechanisms against external influences

— Healthy metabolism, robust vitality

How to Strengthen the Life Principle of the Triple Heater Meridian

The Wheel of Life

Draw a circle and divide it into eight pieces of the same size, like a cake. Your wheel of life is now before you. Allocate each piece of the cake to an area of your life. The following areas should definitely be represented:

- Health – body
- Family – love – relationship
- Friendships – relationships to the people in your environment
- Work
- Finance
- Leisure – relaxation – fun
- Personal development – finding meaning – self-actualisation

Choose an eighth point representing a further important aspect of your life. And then ask yourself the following question: How do I rate my contentment in each area of my life? The maximum possible contentment is 100%. Be honest! This exercise is about taking a sober inventory. Colour in each piece of your cake according to the percentage you've allocated to it: 100% satisfaction means that the colour fills the entire piece, all the way to its outer edge; 0% would remain blank. Now look at your wheel of life. Is it nice and round and running smoothly? Or is it all lopsided because there are too many different grades of contentment? The triple heater is the authority that ensures balance. To strengthen your triple heater, choose the two areas with the lowest percentage and draft a plan to improve your contentment in these two areas over the next month.

Self-Regulation

The triple heater meridian is mindful that we don't get out of balance. However, on the parquet floor of our life, we tend to slip on our feelings. Our emotions cause us to lose our poise easily. However, managing our emotional life is an art that can certainly be learned. This is best done at home. Look for a comfortable place and relax. Bring to mind a situation that happened over the past few days which really rattled your emotions. Try to remember and relive this situation as vividly as you can, while at the same time remaining in the role of an observer. Reflect on the following questions: Where exactly in your body do you feel the emotion you had in that situation? How does it feel in different areas of your body? What kind of thoughts do these feelings bring up? How do they change your breathing, your heart rate? And then, with awareness, take your breath and your focus to precisely the area of your body where your emotion is burning the strongest. Deepen your breathing, relax the affected area until the emotion has calmed down. Bring awareness to the thought that you are not at the mercy of your emotions, that you can manage them. Practise this technique until you are able to regulate yourself to the extent that you can stay calm even during confrontations. Practise until you manage to become aware of the rolling train of your emotions but no longer feel the habitual need to jump on.

The Pathway of the Triple Heater Meridian

The triple heater meridian begins at Triple Heater 1 on the little-finger side of the ring finger, at the corner of the nail. It follows the side of the ring finger to the back of the hand, traversing a depression between the fourth and fifth metacarpal bones. It continues in the groove between these two bones towards the wrist. On the wrist, distal to the head of the ulna, is the point Triple Heater 4.

From Triple Heater 4, the meridian courses along the midline between the ulna and radius. Two thumb-widths along from Triple Heater 4 is Triple Heater 5. The meridian continues further along the midline of the forearm to the elbow, which it crosses between the protrusion of the distal end of the humerus (lateral epicondyle) and the tip of the elbow (olecranon) to reach Triple Heater 10, located in a clearly palpable depression above the olecranon.

The further pathway of the meridian ascends the outer head of the triceps to the posterior border of the deltoid and continues in a groove alongside this muscle to Triple Heater 14, found in the posterior of the two depressions on the deltoid which become apparent below the top of the shoulder when the arm is abducted. From Triple Heater 14, the meridian courses along the spine of the scapula to reach Triple Heater 15, located on a line approximately a thumb-width below the highest point of the trapezius, halfway along the distance between the shoulder and the spine. The meridian then follows the ascending part of the trapezius along a line that courses towards the prominent bony protuberance on the temporal bone, the mastoid process. This is the location of Triple Heater 17. The meridian now contours along the hairline around the ear to Triple Heater 21, which is in a depression in front of the ear on the upper border of the jaw angle. This depression can be palpated when the mouth is slightly open. From Triple Heater 21, the meridian continues towards the eyebrow, where we find Triple Heater 23, the last point on the meridian, in a depression next to the outer end of the eyebrow.

Key Areas of the Triple Heater Meridian

Ears

The triple heater meridian perfectly circles the ear, which is the organ essential for our equilibrium. The ear registers our movements in all three dimensions. Its function is crucial for maintaining a stable sense of our body. Balance and stability, in turn, are the core functions of the triple heater. While being equally sensitive and receptive to any disturbances or changes, its tasks extend to our entire body. In order to fulfil its duties, the triple heater has to be able to listen well so that it can pick up even the most subtle voices of discontent. A key point in this respect is Triple Heater 21, *er men* or 'Ear Gate'. Are we more focussed on listening to the outside world? Or are we also listening to what's going on inside us? Are we deaf towards our own emotions and needs? Are we hard of hearing when our inner voice pipes up? Triple Heater 21 can be used for all kinds of ear problems.

A further important point near the ear is Triple Heater 17, *yi feng* or 'Wind Screen'. Triple Heater 17 not only protects us from the climatic factor wind but generally strengthens our defences against all external influences. This point helps us to keep our balance in the face of gossip-mongering and rumours, which can easily cause stress and tension, especially in the neck and shoulders – in other words, along the further pathway of the triple heater meridian. Triple Heater 17 encourages us to guide our perception towards the interior and lend an ear to ourselves.

Forearm

When we walk through life with open arms, we display the point Pericardium 6, *nei guan* or 'Inner Gate', to our environment. Or we can cross our arms, showing the world the point Triple Heater 5, *wai guan* or 'Outer Pass'. Do we want to embrace others? Or do we want to protect ourselves? While the pericardium meridian is more concerned with matters of the heart, the triple heater is our interface with the outside world, ensuring that everything that is supposed to stay away does indeed stay away. Undesirable influences are supposed to bounce off as manifested in the point Triple Heater 6, *zhi gou* or 'Branch Ditch'. Either point can be used to strengthen the defences of the triple heater. Or to expel any undesirable influences that have managed to enter our system already. To achieve this, it's necessary to open the outer gate. In its capacity as fire point, Triple Heater 6 is an excellent choice to drain the heat that can arise due to inner friction and grinding.

The Triple Heater Meridian: Key Points

- Associated element: Fire element
- Quality: Yang
- Time on the organ clock: 9pm–11pm
- Animal quality: Pig
- Partner meridian: Pericardium meridian
- Twinned meridian: Gallbladder meridian
- Opposite meridian: Spleen meridian

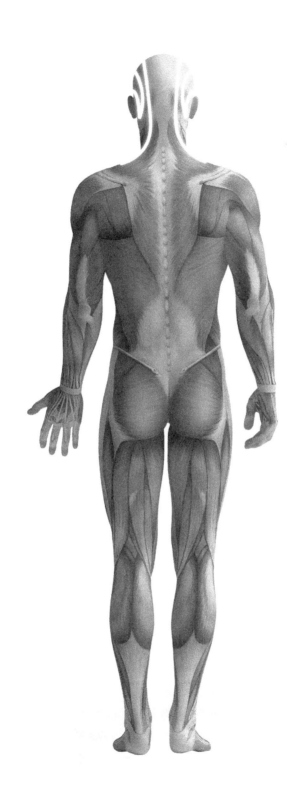

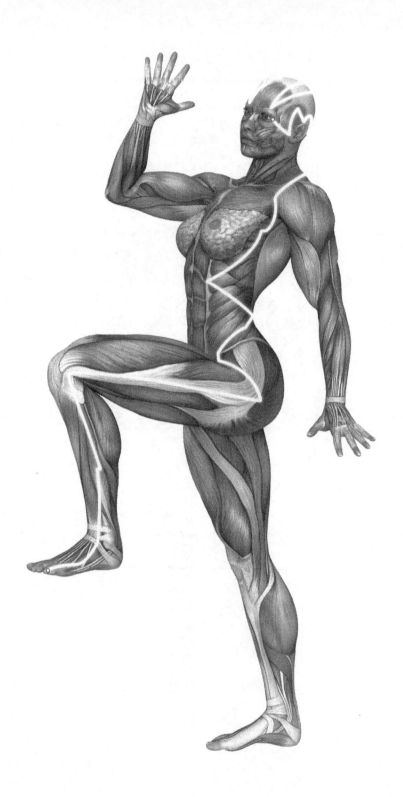

Chapter 15

The Gallbladder Meridian

The Determined General

Questions for the Gallbladder Meridian

- Do I make decisions quickly and without hesitation?
- Am I good at taking on responsibilities?
- Am I resilient?
- Am I able to act in a determined and decisive manner?
- Am I consistent?
- Am I able to listen to my head and trust my gut feeling in equal measure?
- Are my emotions and my thoughts acting in concert?
- Am I able to take a risk?
- Am I able to show courage and fortitude in critical situations?
- Am I able to delegate and put others in charge?
- Am I able to take time out and let go?
- Am I stubborn and persistent?
- Do I find it hard to accept criticism and feedback?

The Life Principle of the Gallbladder Meridian

Someone has to take responsibility. Whatever it may be, the gallbladder has to account for it. In TCM, the gallbladder is often referred to as the body's general. The general decides. He is ultimately responsible for what happens or doesn't happen. A very big task for a very small organ. The pathway of the gallbladder meridian is the longest in our entire body. Starting at the eyes, it controls the lateral aspects of the body all the way down to the toes. Left, right, above, below, the gallbladder meridian is everywhere, getting a sorely needed view of everything that's going on. Its life principle is about making clear and conscious decisions for the benefit of the entire body. The gallbladder leads, determines and takes responsibility. In a nutshell: without the gallbladder meridian, we would flutter through life like a leaf in the wind. We would be at the mercy of random influences and be unable or unwilling to put up any resistance.

What distinguishes General Gallbladder is his determination. He doesn't hesitate, he doesn't procrastinate. Or does he? When the life principle of the gallbladder meridian is only poorly developed, then it's not about making decisions. Rather, it's about endlessly pondering pros and cons, about mulling over every possibility, however trivial it may be. The dominant behaviour is of a rather anxious and timid nature. People like that live life in the hope that the need for making a decision will be taken away from them, by others, by the turn of events, by the passing of time or simply by fate. But if you don't decide yourself, others will do it for you. And if you don't determine what you want, others will determine this for you. The responsibility is taken out of your hands, which means you have to take what you're given. Sometimes this can be pretty bitter, just like bile, which may rise up when you're not satisfied with the conditions around you. But before you start to breathe fire and brimstone without there being a real need for it, you should take back the responsibility that is your due. This, too, is a decision.

A well-developed life principle of the gallbladder meridian knows that it is capable of taking the helm and determining its course. It knows that it is able to respond to the challenges life throws at it. And that's at the core of it all: to take responsibility for ourselves, to be responsible for our life, consistently and uncom- promisingly. Of course, this requires a lot of courage and fortitude because there will always be difficult decisions to make. A good general strides ahead fearlessly; he doesn't know what it means to be afraid. He does what needs to be done; he takes initiative. At each crossroads, big or small, we need our General Gallbladder to show us the direction and set the agenda; otherwise, we would stay put until we turned to stone. And if there is one organ that is susceptible to disorders involving stones, it's the gallbladder.

A good general is fully aware that he cannot and must not achieve everything on his own. One flipside of the gallbladder's life principle is exaggerated responsibility. The gallbladder is quick to raise its hand when there is a load to be carried, either professionally or privately. It likes to meddle and seize things. Of course, the gallbladder does well with pressure and big tasks – after all, it's a general. But this also makes it susceptible to being overburdened as well as overwhelmed, so much so that it ends up feeling responsible for everything while forgetting about itself, until it eventually breaks down under its big loads and all the responsibility. When there is stress and burnout, the gallbladder will have its fingers in the various pies.

A healthy gallbladder meridian, on the other hand, knows its limits and is able to delegate. It is happy to grant responsibility to others. Even though it has a tendency towards being a maverick, it is aware that teamwork is necessary to face truly big challenges. Behind every good general are equally good officers. There are two meridians the gallbladder likes to cooperate with particularly closely: those of the kidney and liver. The kidney meridian stands for our potential, for who we truly are. The liver meridian develops this into a vision, the big masterplan of our life. And the gallbladder realises it with determination, responsibility, courage and conviction. That is its task.

The Gallbladder Meridian and the Body

Left, Right, Rigidity and Stubbornness

The pathway of the gallbladder meridian begins at the eyes and continues to the ears and, by zigzagging on the sides of the head, down to the occipital musculature. Our two most important sensory organs – our ears and our eyes – are therefore under the direct remit of the gallbladder meridian, and they contribute considerably to its ability to stay on top of things. Since the gallbladder also governs our lateral mobility, it allows us to turn our head, to look left and right, to listen to the left and to the right, and to take in the entire surrounding space with all the information contained therein. The gallbladder, as general, needs this overview and the information he gathers as a basis for well-considered decisions.

After all, it is believed that we take between 20,000 and 100,000 decisions every day. This begins in the morning. The alarm clock rings. Should we get up or stay in bed or press the snooze-button? It continues from there. Have a look at the phone first or do some yoga or begin the day with a coffee? Yes? No? Maybe? Including the usual morning routine, decisions such as breakfast and what to wear, we've made several hundred decisions before we have even left the house. Most of them are taken incredibly quickly and unconsciously because they're trivial and inconsequential. But that doesn't apply to all decisions; some are serious and will have far-reaching consequences. That's where the life principle of the gallbladder meridian kicks in, and the general, due to his overview of the situation and his foresight of what's to come, will set the course for our life.

The actions of a gallbladder with a well-developed life principle are clear and judicious. It considers the pros and cons, it weighs up all the possibilities and alternatives, it chooses the best option, it decides and acts, in a direct and unmediated manner. When it is about crucial life questions, this can sometimes be a difficult process. That's quite simply because even if you try to assess a situation from all angles, you will never manage to cover all variables and all possible consequences that may come in the wake of a hugely important decision. It's precisely this kind of situation where we need the life principle of the gallbladder meridian. Because through insecurity and the fear of making the wrong decision, no decision is made at all. Making a decision also means excluding all options that haven't been chosen. But a weak gallbladder meridian likes to keep its options open. It doesn't want to burn any bridges, lose something or take too big a risk. A good general, however, will decide, no matter what. Because he is brave and knows that no decision is still a decision, and if a decision has to be made, it's better to make it consciously, actively, full speed ahead. It's better to carry the responsibility for something that we have chosen ourselves rather than think up answers for a course of action that was put before us by others.

A poorly developed life principle of the gallbladder meridian, on the other hand, will remain passive; it will tread water and will be consistent in its holding back. This attitude clearly expresses itself along the pathway of the gallbladder meridian. Its energy stagnates, and pressure and tension build up, from the left and right sides, the areas controlled by the gallbladder meridian. This pressure constrains us: we lose our freedom of movement, we're no longer on top of things, we become rigid and stubborn, we freeze and get stuck in many loops. Persistent hesitation, procrastination and delaying are part of our daily agenda. We are unable to take the next or the decisive step; our progress is blocked, as is our body. Our head sits immovably on our shoulders, the back of our neck is as flexible as concrete. The basic approach to life is stiff, stubborn, imperturbable, single-minded, pig-headed. There's a tendency to obstinacy, denial and ignorance, even if such attitudes result in the exacerbation or escalation of the problem at hand. Such people solidify completely, so much so that they develop gallstones, which, in TCM, are considered to be a manifestation of long-term stagnation in the gallbladder meridian. Any input from outside is met with resistance. You don't listen to anybody. You turn away and whistle a tune. Until the pressure of your inflexibility gets so big that you can hear the whistling in your ears. Many ear problems are actually associated with the gallbladder, as are problems that arise from severe tension and inflexibility of the musculoskeletal system.

However, gallbladder-related obstinacy can also have its advantages. When a general makes a decision, he's responsible for the consequences – he, and no one else. That's why it's so helpful to listen mostly to ourselves and not let ourselves be influenced by others. That's because a good portion of stubbornness is the best protection against objections and people who like to throw down the gauntlet of doubt in front of us. This allows us to stick to our goals and not be thrown off course from our chosen path. We don't let ourselves be swayed one way or another; we don't turn into turncoats. In this scenario, the gallbladder meridian provides the necessary stability, and our eyes are directed straight ahead rather than darting from side to side. Unyielding. Strong. Determined in the extreme, like a general with a clear goal and a clear vision.

When the life principle of the gallbladder meridian is well integrated, there is a fruitful relationship between flexibility and tenacity, between focus on detail and a wider overview. You're able to look to the sides, look around you, listen to other people, consider their opinions and yet make your own decisions. You don't hesitate. You act.

Stiff occiput and hips, limited range of motion, high muscle tone, muscular tension (back of the neck, shoulders), biliary colic, gallstones, tinnitus...

Bias and Coordination

Coordination is one of the essential tasks of the gallbladder meridian. A good general has to make sure that all troops act in accordance with each other; otherwise, there will be chaos and disagreements, and it will be difficult to pursue a particular direction, which is a further aspect of the gallbladder's life principle. To advance successfully, all units have to act in concert. The gallbladder meridian not only governs the sides of the body, but its pathway also connects above and below. An imbalance of the gallbladder meridian will therefore weaken its capacity for coordination. Left, right, above, below – interactions are no longer fine-tuned, and some areas may become completely disconnected. In such cases, it's certainly not possible to speak about graceful movements. The body no longer forms a unified entity. The shoulders have no connection with the hips, nor do the arms and the legs, and the head has no idea what the feet are up to. People like that seem to act somewhat woodenly. TCM assigns the gallbladder meridian to the wood element, which loses its natural flexibility when out of balance. Based on the pathway of the gallbladder meridian, this imbalance also has a strong influence on the brain. After all, nearly half of the acupuncture points on the gallbladder meridian are located on the head – a further area this meridian has to coordinate.

No matter whether we reflect on something or try to make a decision, both rational and emotional components play a central role in our thinking and acting. Our brain comprises two halves, each of which has a certain focal aspect. The right half of the brain controls intuition, creativity and emotions. It deals with parallel processing of the information it receives, thus keeping an eye on the bigger picture. It is the birthplace of our imagination. The left half of the brain processes information consecutively and in a certain order. This is important for speaking, reading, writing and arithmetic; it's of benefit for logic. The left half of the brain stands for what we commonly refer to as thinking. The right half of the brain is the department for big emotions and coherence. Both halves of the brain together function as a system in which they work in close cooperation. The right half of the brain designs a dream; the left half implements it. Imagination requires logic, and logic requires imagination. Otherwise there will be bias.

There are the following classic archetypes. On the one hand, there is the dreamer who makes the best of things but finds it hard to get a foothold in a world dominated by rules and structures. On the other hand, there's the bone-dry analyst lacking any spontaneous emotion. Together, the two could form a very fruitful partnership, complementing and inspiring each other. But each on its own is a bit of a lost and lonely soul. Both these archetypes are dormant within us – in the right and left half of our brain respectively. For the core task of the gallbladder, it's important that they work in unison. A well-integrated life principle of the gallbladder becomes apparent when emotion and analysis are both given equal space.

Decisions based purely on emotions are determined by a plethora of factors, but in particular by previous engrained experiences. Such experiences lead to emotional associations which complicate a distanced and sober analysis of a situation. Conversely, reaching a decision based on purely rational processes will suppress intuition. But this is necessary, especially when it's about finding solutions for complex challenges, which can never be comprehended based on facts alone. For best results, always ask your head as well as your gut feelings. The power of coordination. The power of unity.

If the life principle of the gallbladder meridian is only poorly developed, it can lead to feelings of inner turmoil. The head wants something other than the emotions. The emotions want something other than the head. Inner conflict and divisiveness – a typical gallbladder problem. People are at the mercy of their emotions or their inner analyst, depending on whether they prefer to trust their head or their guts. Due to being excessively biased, they don't have much choice how to react or behave. They are aware that something is missing: the other side.

A one-sided dominance can further lead to many physical problems. It's a question of how the tension in one side relates to the other side. A disharmony in the gallbladder meridian results in instability. We lose our balance, like a tightrope walker losing their poise. This can lead to vertigo and loss of equilibrium. Or the body becomes distorted, with either the hips or the spine affected. That's the root cause leading to further disorders: one-sided problems are attributed primarily to the gallbladder meridian – for example, back pain, wear and tear of the hip joints, and sciatica, but also migraine-type headaches or strokes.

A well-integrated life principle of the gallbladder meridian provides balance, equilibrium and suppleness, and it also makes sure that all aspects of our personality are interacting in a supportive and fine-tuned manner: head and guts, left and right, above and below. There's a clear-cut course. That's what General Gallbladder stands for.

SYMPTOMS ASSOCIATED WITH THE GALLBLADDER MERIDIAN

One-sided symptoms and problems, hip and back disorders, spinal disorders, sciatica, coordination problems, balance problems, vertigo...

The Gallbladder Meridian and the Psyche

Hesitation, Procrastination and Anger

That a general likes to make decisions and push forward is obvious. But it's not always like that. A poorly developed life principle of the gallbladder meridian does the opposite. The general hesitates. He plays for time. He distinguishes himself by putting things on the back burner. Impending tasks and decisions are postponed. The more important and challenging, the greater the delay. This is procrastination, an increasingly pervasive phenomenon. *Pro* means 'for' and *crastinum* means 'tomorrow'. We decide not to decide. At least not today. Nor tomorrow. Even if we finally manage to make a decision, we will doubt it the next moment and often abandon it again. Instead, we prefer to occupy ourselves with alternative tasks, which lead us to believe that we are busy and also guarantee distraction. Pleasant activities rather than unpleasant effort. Cleaning rather than tax return. Facebook rather than textbook. The moment is more inviting than the future.

A weakened gallbladder meridian, on the other hand, lacks orientation and focus on the next step in the direction of a more distant goal. The causes of this are many. Often, the kidney meridian has a finger in the pie. It provides the inner motives and the necessary motivation. But if the kidney meridian isn't strong enough, it is inhibited by the fear of challenge, of failure, or the fear of reconciling our ideal with reality. A disharmony of the gallbladder meridian is often expressed in fundamentally insecure and fearful attitudes. It takes the courage of a general to grab pending tasks by the horns and get them done. It requires clarity to set relevant priorities and to consciously distance oneself from tempting alternative options. Having a weak gallbladder certainly doesn't help. A weak gallbladder finds it difficult to focus; it prefers to distract itself. This has to do with the pathway of its meridian.

The gallbladder governs not only the sides of the body but also an important extraordinary meridian, the girdling vessel, which circles the middle of the body like a belt or girdle. By governing the sides of the body and by means of the girdle, the gallbladder meridian holds together the body, as well as the emotions and the mind, like a vase gathering together a bunch of flowers. Without a vase, the bunch would fall apart. A weak gallbladder, and the body falls apart. The body, concentration, attention: everything gets wide, soft, and dissolves. The result is instability, insecurity and doubt. The joints are hypermobile, the tissue weak and without tone, especially on the belly since the pull of the belt is missing. The neck turns as easily as a weathervane – General Gallbladder has become General Turncoat, preferring to have the wind at his back, lacking the willpower to face the wind. It gets difficult for you to set a course and find your way. No wonder that decisions are put on the back burner. You're completely out of your depth.

The problem is that in such a situation we are often far from exhausting all our options. We lack purpose, single-mindedness and courage. Being courageous means pulling ourselves together, getting our act together. A well-developed life principle of the gallbladder has the capacity to do precisely that. It supports from both the sidelines and the centre. This sharpens the focus and consolidates the energy. Ultimately, it can even lead to tunnel vision, being like a general who is hell-bent on getting his way. We are on a permanent collision course, even though the one thing we can't bear is a collision. Due to our narrow-mindedness, we tend to be unable to take in anything further or give anything out. We are immune to any feedback from our environment, likely responding to it by spitting bile and poison. Criticism is not allowed, and admitting mistakes is impossible. Deafness towards any feedback makes it hard for us to change course, even if our course is set towards a precipice.

Once again, it's all about balance. A well-integrated life principle of the gallbladder meridian holds the reins neither too tightly nor too loosely. It's able to spur itself on when this is appropriate. By the same token, it's able to adjust its course if and when required.

Taking Responsibility and Delegating

The gallbladder is the meridian of responsibility. If responsibility refers to acting independently within a given framework, it will lead to a feeling of freedom which the gallbladder appreciates so much. However, taking responsibility isn't always a voluntary decision; often it is transferred to us, whether we like it or not. Or it can be imposed on us by life's circumstances. Often the weight of the burden is too big for us. Then responsibility won't lead to freedom but will limit us and, over time, wear us down. For General Gallbladder, it is therefore important to be able to delegate.

However, a gallbladder with a poorly developed life principle will find it difficult to relinquish tasks and responsibilities since the general is worried about his position as leader. Delegating could be interpreted as weakness. It could lead to things being done differently from how you think they should be done. Therefore, you prefer to do things yourself, also because you're convinced that you can do them better and faster. Furthermore, part of the general's character is his predilection for power, for which he is more than willing to pay a price. He who acts has power. He who acts a lot will be overpowering. Like no other meridian, the gallbladder meridian is prone to exaggeration when it comes to taking responsibility. This predestines people with good gallbladder energy to leadership roles. The other side of the coin is that the gallbladder meridian is susceptible to overburdening itself as the combination of a sense of responsibility, determination and obstinacy knows no limits: working till you drop, considering recreation time as highly overvalued and leisure as a sign of lacking consistency. You always want to be at the front line and win. That's the only way you know how. You become a slave to General Gallbladder. It's impossible to let go and relax, even if that was perfectly possible.

A gallbladder with a well-integrated life principle, on the other hand, will recognise its limits. It doesn't mind delegating and sharing tasks without instantly descending into an identity crisis. It can delegate without questioning its entire existence. A good general understands keeping himself in the background and sending others to the front line should they be better suited. These are people who understand how to promote and encourage others instead of constantly being demanding. They are cognisant about the importance of pooling resources when it comes to important tasks and goals. This ensures efficiency and efficacy. Ultimately, this is also about self-responsibility: the general has to maintain his strength. A disordered gallbladder meridian tends to forget about balancing its job with relaxation. It often puts health problems on the back burner because it doesn't find the time to deal with them. For the gallbladder to stay balanced, it is therefore important to cultivate noble idleness and grant itself breaks at consistent intervals. Even a general is entitled to some holiday. A gallbladder with a well-developed life principle feels perfectly confident taking time out. It acts towards its self as responsibly as it does towards its other roles.

Signs of an Imbalanced and Balanced Gallbladder Meridian

Signs of an Imbalanced Gallbladder Meridian

- Difficulties with decision making, hesitant, procrastinating, timid

- Insecurity, little courage for taking risks, inhibited
- Difficulties with pulling oneself together and staying focussed
- Little sense of responsibility, not very action-/goal-oriented
- Unstable, uncoordinated, internally conflicted
- Tendency towards overburdening and over-extending oneself, unable to delegate
- Likes to dominate and take over, constantly interfering
- Tendency to back pain, tension in the shoulders and the occiput, balance problems, tinnitus...

Signs of a Balanced Gallbladder Meridian

- Pronounced sense of responsibility, able to cope with stress
- Decisiveness, determination, fearlessness
- Stays on top of things, quick grasp, quick to implement a decision
- Balance between head and gut, between thinking and feeling
- Capacity to pursue long-term goals, no procrastination, not easily distracted
- Healthy balance between delegating and acting
- Good at coordinating

How to Strengthen the Life Principle of the Gallbladder Meridian

Deciding Like a Samurai

'Never take more than seven breaths when you need to make a decision' is the advice given by samurais. Try it. Our ability to make quick decisions is like a muscle that can be trained. Begin with small decisions. If you start jogging, you won't start with running the distance of a marathon. In our everyday life, there are plenty of opportunities to strengthen our decision-making muscle. Set yourself the goal of making at least two decisions per day within the time it takes for seven breaths, without hesitating or wavering.

Best suited are challenges with few consequences yet requiring to be pondered. Finish the process with a clear decision. Simply do it. And then stand by it.

Delegating Responsibility

Find a task for which you consider yourself the best and most suitable person. Then delegate this task to somebody else. In the meantime, take responsibility for yourself and do something that you really enjoy, something that recharges your batteries and regenerates you. Don't meddle and don't try to check whether your quality standards and your values are being met. Concentrate on the essential – on yourself. You may be surprised: the world keeps on turning.

The Pathway of the Gallbladder Meridian

The gallbladder meridian begins half a thumb-width lateral to the outer corner of the eye, the location of the point Gallbladder 1. The meridian then courses towards the ear, traversing the cheekbone as it does so, until it reaches Gallbladder 2, situated directly anterior to the attachment of the ear, in a depression that forms when the mouth is open. From there, the meridian ascends towards the forehead, where Gallbladder 4 is located within the hairline. Its further pathway sees the meridian returning to the ear and curving around it to reach Gallbladder 12, which can be found a little below and behind the tip of the prominent bony protrusion on the temporal bone (mastoid process). From Gallbladder 12, the meridian runs laterally across the skull to Gallbladder 14, located a thumb-width above the centre of the eyebrow. In a wide arc, it's back across the skull to Gallbladder 20, situated at the lower occipital border, in a depression between the two distinctly palpable muscle strands of the sternocleidomastoid and the trapezius.

From Gallbladder 20, the meridian continues in a groove between the lateral and posterior neck muscles to Gallbladder 21, located on the anterior border of the trapezius.

The next section of the meridian can be found on the front of the body, between the pectoralis major and the deltoid. It then veers laterally to Gallbladder 22 on the lateral chest, more precisely in the fourth intercostal space, below the anterior armpit fold. Here the meridian does a little sidestep, by coursing a thumb-width towards the front (Gallbladder 23), before continuing in the direction of Gallbladder 24 in the seventh intercostal space. From there, it follows the contours of the rib towards the back and to the lower border of the twelfth (floating) rib, the location of Gallbladder 25. At this point, the meridian once again changes direction, traversing the waist to reach Gallbladder 26, which can be found on the lateral midline of the body at the level of the navel. The meridian then courses to the anterior bony projection of the hip bone (the anterior superior iliac spine). Gallbladder 27 is located half a thumb-width in front of it, while Gallbladder 28 is another half thumb-width below Gallbladder 27.

The meridian now continues over the side of the pelvis to Gallbladder 30, located in a depression behind the greater trochanter. From here, the meridian follows the gluteus maximus. Once it reaches the thigh, it courses down the midline of its lateral aspect, along a distinctly strengthened band of fascia, right where one would normally find the seam of someone's trousers. From there, it's further down the leg, crossing the outside of the knee, to Gallbladder 34, located in a depression anterior and inferior to the head of the fibula. On the lower leg, the meridian follows the fibula and curves anteriorly past the lateral malleolus to Gallbladder 40, which can be found in a marked depression anterior and inferior to the lateral malleolus. From Gallbladder 40, the meridian courses over the back of the foot between the fourth and fifth metatarsal bones and reaches its terminal point, Gallbladder 44, on the outer corner of the nail of the fourth toe.

Key Areas of the Body

Head and Occiput

No other meridian dominates the head like the gallbladder meridian. Its pathway clearly mirrors its tasks. It connects the two sensory organs most important for spatial perception: the eyes and the ears. They ensure foresight as well as keeping an overview. This requires the head to be mobile. One of the most important cranial points is Gallbladder 12, *wan gu* or 'Completion Bone', located directly at the insertion of the large muscle belly of the sternocleidomastoid, which tilts the head to the side and is also responsible for lateral rotation. The point Gallbladder 20, *feng chi* or 'Wind Pool', can be found in the area governed by the trapezius, a further important muscle controlling the head and the occiput. When the gallbladder meridian is tense, this will impair the range of motion in this area, and we get stiff-necked and stubborn. We'll have had it quickly 'up to here' (which is usually somewhere high up on the neck) when others don't agree with us. This limited range of motion is also reflected in our mentality as it limits our outlook on life. What remains is tunnel vision, looking straight ahead. A weakness in this area, on the other hand, results in us turning our head depending on where the wind is coming from. We easily adopt the opinions and wishes of others since we're lacking stability.

Twenty out of a total of 44 gallbladder points are located on the head. The direction of flow is from above to below. The density of the points there, in connection with the way it zig-zags on the lateral aspect of the head, makes it particularly susceptible to congestion and stagnation. Many symptoms in the head are therefore related to the gallbladder meridian.

Waist and Hips

The waist is dominated by the girdle vessel, which can be considered a branch of the gallbladder meridian. The girdle vessel holds the middle together; it stabilises our centre and provides us with strength. It supports us in the same manner as the gallbladder meridian supports the kidneys and the lumbar spine in this area. The point Gallbladder 25, *jing men* or 'Capital Gate', is located on the lower end of the twelfth rib. It is also the alarm point of the kidneys. The kidneys stand for our potential, given to us at birth for us to fulfil. The kidneys stand for the 'capital' within us. Gallbladder 25 gives us direct access not only to this capital but to everything contained therein. The kidney meridian needs the gallbladder meridian, and the gallbladder meridian needs the kidney meridian. After all, how are we supposed to let our potential unfold other than with determination, courage and clear decisions? If we fail to fulfil our potential, alarm bells will start ringing in the kidneys as we aren't exhausting our capacities. This also limits our range of motion, and we circulate through life within a very small perimeter. The point Gallbladder 30, *huan tiao* or 'Jumping Round', expresses this perfectly. How big is the area we cover with our (life) circle? Or do we remain in one spot, stuck in just one place?

Gallbladder 30 governs the hip, particularly the range of motion to the sides. When we find ourselves at a crossroads, Gallbladder 30 is the authority that guides our decision for turning left or right. The lack of clarity in what we want and our insecurity or timidity for asserting our will and our wishes block the progress on our life path. Gallbladder 25 and Gallbladder 26 have a strong connection based on their function. When the life principle of the gallbladder meridian is well developed, this results in good balance between stability and mobility in the hip and waist. A weakness in that area can lead to instability and hypermobility of the lumbar spine. The vertebrae can shift easily, the spine loses its shape, the discs begin to slide, and the hip joint is susceptible to dislocation. But too much tension can also be a cause of many problems. Lack of suppleness makes the spine susceptible to strain as well as wear and tear, and also to stiffness and lack of mobility.

The Gallbladder Meridian: Key Points

- Associated element: Wood element
- Quality: Yang
- Time on the organ clock: 11pm–1am
- Animal quality: Rat
- Partner meridian: Liver meridian
- Twinned meridian: Triple heater meridian
- Opposite meridian: Heart meridian

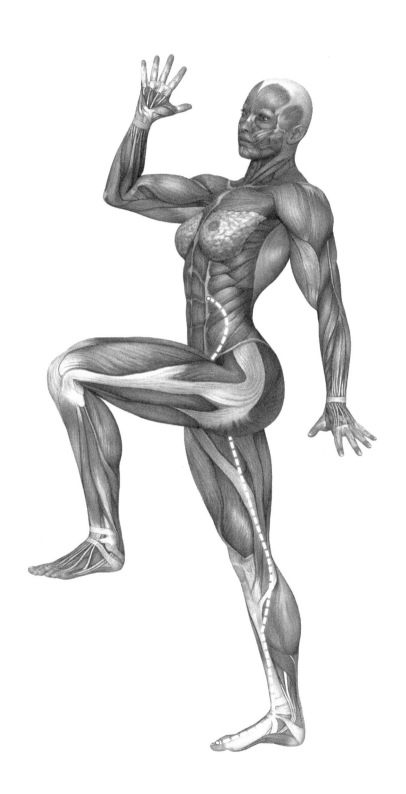

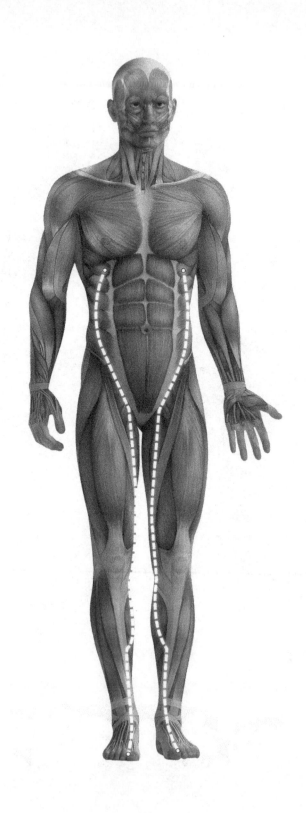

Chapter 16

The Liver Meridian

The Creative Free Spirit

Questions for the Liver Meridian

- Do I have dreams and visions?
- Do I have a masterplan for my innermost wishes?
- Am I able to be creative?
- Do I find it easy to take on new perspectives?
- Am I able to approach things with the necessary zest and appropriate assertiveness?
- Do I have a constructive relationship with my aggression?
- Am I able to give my emotions free rein?
- Do I have the confidence to be angry or show my anger?
- Am I able to respond flexibly towards unforeseen events?
- Am I able to adapt well to new circumstances?
- Am I physically as well as mentally supple and agile?

The Life Principle of the Liver Meridian

The liver is the body's organ of spring. It wants to grow, evolve, move, and it wants to do all that without constraints. The liver is about big adventures and great deeds. The liver meridian is the last of the twelve meridians to come into its power. Its breakthrough occurs around puberty, at the time when a young person is cutting their umbilical cord to their parents. It's the beginning of their journey towards autonomy, towards shaping their own existence. The life principle of the liver meridian is about crafting the best possible vision based on the essence of all other meridians – a vision that is tailored to a person's potential – and tackling this vision with dynamic creativity. The liver meridian stands for our deepest dreams, for freedom and intensity.

To this end, the liver needs two personality traits in particular: aggression and flexibility. The word 'aggression' comprises two Latin words, *ad* and *gradus*, which quite simply means to approach something with equally firm and determined steps, to really make a go of something. The energy of spring doesn't like waiting or being held back. It is loaded with expectations and wants to go about its task, which is to show itself in all its glory and all its colours. When the life principle of the liver is well developed, aggression can become a tool that is consciously used for realising plans and ideas rather than just dreaming about them.

But when the liver's life principle is blocked, there may well be much dreaming, but nothing comes of it. This is frustrating since 'should've, could've, would've' has never made a flower blossom, even when spring is exploding all around. In such a scenario, aggression will certainly come into play too at some point, but rather in the form of rage. This is because people like that are loaded and tense, like a bud. All a bud wants is to burst open, but it just isn't managing it. What we are left with is a frustrated liver instead of a lovely scent. Your environment will notice this. You turn sour; you get cross with others, cross with yourself, cross with life, because reality and your idea of what reality should be like are miles apart. The energy of spring is frozen. And along with it, the free flow of liver energy is stagnant as well. This will render a person stiff and rigid, and, as a result, the liver meridian will get even more cross since it loves flexibility and adaptability.

Flexibility is very much an attitude. It's the spring in our head. Among the organs, the liver is the creative free spirit, bubbling with ideas. Everything is possible. When the life principle of the liver is well developed, you're great at thinking laterally and outside the box. You have solutions to problems that haven't even occurred yet. Inventive and creative thinking, as well as the ability to perform several mental splits simultaneously, results in quick responses and adaptability. New situations are seen as opportunities that allow us to grow. The liver loves a good challenge. However, when the liver is weak, a challenge will break it. That's because a blocked liver meridian is as flexible as an iron rod in permafrost. Such people will perceive every change as a personal threat because they are unable or unwilling to adapt. Out of fear of the unknown or fear of growth, what is known becomes cemented, even if it sucks the will to live out of the body. People get completely stuck – professionally, in their relationships, in their behavioural patterns. They'd rather tear themselves up inside than tear the world apart. There's no fun at all; being cross is the order of the day. Like that, life simply isn't enjoyable.

With a harmonious liver meridian you can experience life like a warm spring day, which magically brings a smile to your face. Open the doors, have fun; get the horses out of the stable and gallop away at full tilt into the big wide world, full of adventures. Give yourself free rein and enjoy yourself.

The Liver Meridian and the Body

Looking Back, Looking Ahead

The liver and heart meridians both have a direct connection with the eyes. The heart meridian sees in order to recognise and to understand. The liver meridian sees what has been and what could be in the future. The heart meridian represents insights. The liver meridian represents looking back and looking ahead. What have I experienced, and how does this affect the way I see things? How could my life develop if only I had enough confidence to dream big without any constraints? What is my vision? The liver likes to develop the kind of positive outlook that engenders an atmosphere of new beginnings, a spring-like energy. The liver wants to grow, it wants to move. It is able to manoeuvre us out of situations in which we feel bogged down and stuck. It knows how to set sail for new territories. But in order to succeed, the liver has to get rid of unnecessary baggage first...

It's not just in Western medicine that the liver is considered a formidable storage organ. TCM describes the liver as the reservoir of blood. The blood, in turn, also has storage functions. It is the carrier and anchor of our consciousness. Together, the liver and the blood form a kind of internal hard drive for our memories, referred to as the *hun*. The *hun* stands for the aspect of our consciousness that stores memory. The *hun* partially represents the Western concept of the subconscious. It stores everything we experience as images and feelings. It is like a photo album of our life story. How far does our story go back? That's a matter of opinion. Some people believe our biography begins with our birth, others see our beginning at the time of conception, and then there are those who consider reincarnation not as a philosophical construct but as a reality. The *hun* is therefore also referred to as the 'wandering soul'. It carries impressions and experiences from one life to the next. Whichever it may be, the *hun* has a considerable influence on how we see and experience the world around us.

If we let the *hun* take the helm, we'll be entirely at the mercy of being controlled by our subconscious. We will be governed by habitual patterns from the past. Past experiences will determine how we see the present. To some extent, that's perfectly normal, of course; it's part of the learning curve of our life. But depending on the content of the hard drive, it can be a very limiting and curtailing factor, and significantly impair the leeway for manoeuvre so important for the liver meridian. The *hun*, as a kind of hard drive, may contain programs that favour behavioural routines and thus boycott our plans for growth and evolving. We tend to react without reflection and lose our ability for conscious action. We are no longer the captain of the ship that's our life; we're a mere stowaway. We rattle off the same program, again and again, like a stuck record player. The same habits, the same thoughts, the same answers, the same problems, over and over. No change, no flexibility, but always lots of emotions since the associated memories and feelings are constantly aroused. We repeat the same things: You remind me of my father, you remind me of my mother, you remind me of my ex, this reminds me of my childhood, this reminds me of what happened last year, this reminds me of this or that or such and such, and so on and so forth. We are unable to see what could be;

we only ever see what has been. We arbitrarily subject ourselves to the wind and waves of bygone years. Sentimentality becomes our default setting, and this can happen even in young people.

When the life principle of the liver is only poorly developed, the liver finds it hard to process the residual waste of the *hun* and to take on a more creative view about its future. It will be unable to come up with big dreams and inspiring visions because it is so busy with all it has lived through in its past. Instead of spring, there is autumn or winter in the head. Stagnation instead of expansion and development. Short-sightedness instead of vision. The mood corresponds to this state of affairs: it's bad and you feel liverish. Aggression, a quality associated with the liver, is not able to discharge and stagnates within. We turn into a powder keg that is getting increasingly full. We turn into a dangerous load, which not only causes suffering in those around us, but also affects our eyes, which are associated with the liver. The pressure on the overflowing storage consciousness (the *hun*) will ultimately lead to raised pressure within, leading to raised intraocular pressure. When there is so much pressure, it takes only the tiniest spark to cause a powerful explosion: one wrong word, one wrong glance, one wrong reaction at the wrong time can result in emotional outbursts of great intensity. The output is completely out of proportion to the input. This is the classic choleric temperament. The red mist comes down on the liver meridian. It is easily inflamed, and this includes the eyes. They are liable to be sensitive and susceptible to becoming irritated, with a tendency towards dryness. They strain easily and don't cope well with wind or sunlight. They are energetically weak and thus form a good substrate for many degenerative eye diseases.

If the *hun* doesn't find a way to vent its tension during the day, then it will catch up during the night. Intense dreams with vivid images and strong emotions are a typical feature of a disturbed liver energy. First of all, the residual waste of everyday life will be eliminated – all the impressions that we have gathered and accumulated. Only once this has been taken care of can the next deeper level come to the fore: all the experiences that have been suppressed and have not been consciously dealt with. And when this level has been cleared, we begin to get closer and closer to our *hun* consciousness. Depending on what the *hun* has stored, the night can be a never-ending nightmare or a source of inspiration. Not everything that has accumulated in the *hun* is necessarily bad. During its travels, the wandering soul has learned many things. The *hun* is a source of talents, gifts and aptitudes, which often can't be explained through logic. There are people who learn exotic languages with ease, who feel at home in certain countries even though they've never been there before. There are people who, even as young children, had talents that surpass our imagination. For the *hun*, this isn't magic; it's simply about accessing memories, about getting in touch with the jewels of our personal treasure trove of experience. In the *hun*, liberated from its limiting residual waste, there slumbers a great vision, a big dream. Getting in touch with our visions and dreams brings a shining brightness to our eyes and opens up completely new perspectives.

SYMPTOMS ASSOCIATED WITH THE LIVER MERIDIAN

Sensitive eyes, light sensitivity, susceptibility to eye infections, dry eyes, raised intraocular pressure, short-sightedness, macular degeneration, vivid dreams with lively imagery, disturbed sleep, nightmares, heightened emotional reactions, tendency to sentimentality...

Flexibility and Adaptability

In TCM, one of the main tasks of the liver meridian is to safeguard the free flow of energy. This free flow facilitates bringing into the world what is lying dormant within us by means of a big master-plan. This requires free travel and clear thoroughfares. It requires spaciousness and scope for development, especially in the big joints, since these are responsible for the freedom of movement in our body. When our hips and shoulders are open and flexible, we can move easily and quickly in all directions. We can charge ahead and chase our dreams. This, in turn, requires supple muscles and sinews, which also come under the remit of the liver. Once again, this is about the energetic qualities of spring and the power of growth that goes along with it.

The pathway of the liver meridian controls in particular the adductors on the inner thigh. When the adductors are tight, the range of movement of the hips is impaired. Instead of striding along dynamically on a grand scale so as to take up our space, we scuttle around without making any headway, held back by the taut ropes of our musculature. Instead of spurring on our inner horse, we rein it in. Striding forward takes more energy than necessary. Generally, it's not only the hips that are blocked; there's a build-up of tension in the entire body because the liver's intrinsic spring-like energy can't discharge itself and stagnates, like a river held back by an enormous dam. The pent-up pressure gradually increases the muscle tone in the entire body, and the tendons lose their suppleness. The neck, the back, the shoulders, the chest, the waist – everything hardens, gets stiff and tight. And not just on a physical level.

Our physical mobility as mediated by the liver meridian is a direct mirror image of our mental and emotional flexibility. It's easy to observe this: when we're young and in the spring of our life, we are open, we're brimming with ideas, our imagination knows no bounds. Our physical foundation is soft, smooth and extremely mobile. But once we reach old age, the autumn or winter of our life, we'll have internalised quite fixed views of what life should be like. Change is no longer really welcome. We prefer stability and continuity. At the same time, our mobility is waning, physically, mentally and also emotionally. That's a normal process. However, this can also set in at a much earlier time of our lives if our liver energy wasn't able to evolve properly. Then autumn will come early, even though we're still in the prime of our lives. Winter will settle in our mind, heart and body prematurely. There will be severe tension, and the muscles turn into a corset, with both mobility and flexibility impaired. A build-up of internal pressure will turn us into a pressure cooker that has unlearned how to release its steam so that our head has to take on the function of the pressure valve – migraines galore. In a tight liver meridian, the smallest trigger can make the head throb: a change in the weather, a change in hormone levels or a little bit more stress in the workplace. This often goes hand in hand with high blood pressure because at some point everything is under pressure. Pressure is the opposite of the freedom so beloved by the liver. Pressure also under-mines another of the liver's tasks – its capacity to adapt.

A liver with a well-developed life principle turns us into a succulent green spring branch: strong yet flexible. Full of life yet yielding. Come wind or stress, the branch can bow and bend, without breaking or losing its shape. As soon as the constraining factors are removed, it returns to its original state. The liver meridian allows us to adapt to stress, strain and unforeseen situations, to go with the flow, without losing our identity. Mental, emotional as well as physical elasticity allows us to flow smoothly along the rapids of everyday life, without much frictional loss, without unnecessary waves, without frustration and annoyance. The liver meridian is the meridian providing us with the gift of patience, equanimity and tolerance.

But it doesn't take much to break a dry branch. However, its lack of flexibility will initially cause resistance. Resistance against even the most minimal changes, the least bit of pressure. We feel easily overwhelmed, and in accordance with our liver's concentrated spring energy, we are prone to lashing out angrily and aggressively if confronted with a limitation of our space. Everything is taken personally. Our threshold for feeling frustrated is low; our impatience with ourselves and others is high. A liver meridian with a well-integrated life principle endows us with openness, a readiness for change, mental flexibility. These traits allow us to act calmly, flexibly and successfully even in chaotic situations.

SYMPTOMS ASSOCIATED WITH THE LIVER MERIDIAN

Pressure sensations, feeling tense, feeling constricted, difficulty breathing, impaired mobility, stiffness, joint problems, headaches, migraines, hypertension...

The Liver Meridian and the Psyche

Creativity, Chaos and a Plan

The life principle of the liver meridian, with its predilection for movement, flexibility and spaciousness, stands for creativity. Creativity arises when we allow our thoughts to fly freely. Creativity means to create something, to invent something. It means new ideas, approaches, views, plans and projects. A liver meridian with a well-developed life principle likes to think expansively and without any limitations. In TCM, the liver represents the architect. The lungs are also seen as architects, but they are the architects of the body, while the liver designs the master plan for life. This plan can be generous and spacious. Or it can be tight and pragmatic.

The Latin term *creare* comprises 'to choose' and 'to create'. The crucial questions for the liver meridian are therefore: What can we truly imagine accomplishing in our life? Do we have the courage to think the impossible? Do we acknowledge possibilities and opportunities corresponding to our boldest dreams? Are we able to come up with a plan that brings us closer to our goals? This requires creativity. After all, if your thought processes are always along the same lines, you're clearly travelling along a rut that has been trodden since the year dot. This is a characteristic trait of a disturbed liver meridian: to rely on tried and tested paths, to prefer the well-established low-risk route. Meanwhile, we're staring longingly towards the mountains and summits that we would like to climb, but the fear of the unpredictable nature of such adventures leaves us intimidated and paralysed.

For the life principle of the liver meridian, it's important that creativity and planning go hand in hand. Hence also the inclusion of 'to choose' in the word *creare*. Creativity without a plan can quickly descend into chaos. There may be lots of fanciful ideas floating around our heads, we may be constructing many a castle in the air in cloud cuckoo land, but none is ever built in real life. The architect in us is completely overwhelmed. There are so many concurrent building sites to be looked after that not a single project is ever completed in a meaningful way. There's a tendency to be like the dreamy romantic who wanders the world full of amazement and with big eyes, but never really hacks anything. True to its dynamic nature, an imbalance in the liver meridian can result in us spreading our energy in all directions, while completely and hopelessly scattering ourselves, too. People with a weak liver meridian are susceptible to chaos of any shape or size. There may be a lack of order in their home or in the workplace, or they jump from one job to the next, from one relationship to the next, from one place of residence to the next. You could, of course, see this as a lively and creative way of leading your life. Or as hopelessly chaotic, since stimuli and actions don't follow a coherent plan.

It can also be extremely frustrating for the liver when things don't go according to plan. When we haven't factored in enough leeway but are determined to stick to our plan, even if reality demands something completely different. A strong liver meridian can handle any change of plan and anything unpredictable extremely well, since it is flexible and dynamic and has a creative answer at the ready for each and every challenge. Adapting to new circumstances is no problem at all. But it certainly is for a weak liver. A weak liver will quickly get panicky at the slightest deviation from the plan. There is no wiggle room to allow changes. The liver lacks the ability to think outside the box. We obstinately stick to the path taken, even if it clearly leads into a cul-de-sac, because we don't know how to change course. This can be frustrating. And it also means we continue to underachieve.

A well-developed life principle of the liver is able to bring forth great visions, to make conscious choices and, based on these choices, develop an adequate plan. It ensures that we live our dream rather than dreaming our life.

Growth and Righteous Anger

The life principle of the liver meridian is all about growing and evolving. These processes require space. Without space, nothing can evolve. It's as simple as that. After all, where could you grow to when there are constraints in every direction? Sometimes these constraints are there from the outset. Sometimes our space is taken away from us whether we like it or not. The liver has two options for how to respond: either by adapting or with aggression. We either yield or we reclaim our space, if necessary by banging our fist on the table to defend our territory. Aggression is an extremely dynamic and explosive form of energy. We need to learn how to deal with it. That's the task of the liver meridian, albeit not an easy one.

Dealing with anger is generally not easy. Our good upbringing tends to get in the way. Being nice – always. We bottle up our resentment rather than showing and venting it. When our liver meridian is imbalanced, we quickly feel uneasy, especially when it comes to anger and rage. We hold back and store any resentment or discontent for months, years or even decades: an accumulation of bad moods deep within us. Being disgruntled becomes our life principle. A dormant hatred of everything and anything, including ourselves. Depression instead of aggression. The opposite of the spring-like energy a strong liver meridian stands for. But sometimes, when too much tension has built up, a cleansing thunderstorm is sorely needed. The liver meridian facilitates healthy access to the aggression lying dormant within us. It facilitates a conscious culture of conflict in the knowledge that sometimes we just have to let off steam in order to clear the air of stagnant and suppressed feelings. The following are important questions for the liver meridian: Am I able to express my anger? Am I able to use aggression consciously and free of guilt in order to create my space? Am I able to have an argument when necessary?

Aggression can also be of benefit should bigger hurdles block our growth process. In such a scenario, the liver meridian endows us with assertiveness, the punch and the courage necessary for confrontation. It can give us the energy boost needed for a 'now more than ever' attitude that will carry us on the home stretch. It endows us with the capacity to tenaciously keep up the pursuit of a solution until the problem has been wrestled to the ground, faint and exhausted. A liver with a poorly developed life principle is unable to do that. It prefers to avoid any potential difficulties. It would rather bend over backwards than bend reality to suit its needs. It would rather destroy its dreams than clear the obstacles in its path.

Destroying? This, too, is an aspect of aggression. Sometimes the old has to be destroyed for the new to arise. This can be painful; it can hurt. But if you want to build a new house, you have to pull down the old one first. Yes, this means scorched earth, but scorched earth can be extremely fertile. A well-integrated life principle of the liver meridian isn't afraid of intense changes if they are indeed necessary for following one's vision. Sometimes our lives have to be turned upside down completely to gain new perspectives and insights. And, if required, with the adequate amount of aggression.

Signs of an Imbalanced and Balanced Liver Meridian

Signs of an Imbalanced Liver Meridian

- Inner and outer tension, stiff joints, high muscle tone
- Extremely sensitive to pressure and changes
- Little flexibility and adaptability
- Little motivation, little assertiveness, little punch
- Prone to headaches, migraines, eye problems, menstrual problems...
- Castles in the air and pipe dreams instead of action
- Chaotic, unstructured, getting lost in tasks or people

Signs of a Balanced Liver Meridian

- Much creativity, lots of ideas, great imagination
- Good at planning and implementing
- Physically active and flexible
- Able to respond and adapt quickly
- No fear of resistance or confrontation
- Able to deal positively with conflicts and arguments
- Innovative, always open to uncharted territories, always a step ahead

How to Strengthen the Life Principle of the Liver Meridian

Dream Big

What would it be like if everything were possible for you? What would you do if you suddenly won several millions on the lottery? What would your life look like then? What would you change? Nothing at all? Congratulations! You are already living your vision, of yourself and your life, and you see no reason to change course. However, if that's not the case, take some time out and let your thoughts soar. What are your desires? What are your dreams? Think big – as big as possible! Build your ideal castle in the air and write down what it looks like. Here's the important question for the liver meridian: Have you already taken steps in the direction of your dreams? Yes? No? Why not? And if not, develop a plan. What counts is the general direction. The little activities. Perhaps not everything is possible. But most likely much more than you think.

Get Angry!

When was the last time you shouted really loudly? When did you last bang your fist on the table? When did you last argue passionately and intensely? When have you actively sought a confrontation rather than avoiding it? Conflict management certainly has its place, but nothing releases the energy of the liver meridian as quickly as a proper outburst of anger. Treat yourself to such a cleansing thunderstorm, consciously and once a week. And if you are worried you will hurt someone, scream while you drive, beat up a cushion or kick a punchbag. Let it all out, no holds barred.

The Pathway of the Liver Meridian

The liver meridian begins with Liver 1 on the outside of the big toe, at the corner of the nail, from where it courses towards Liver 2, located between the first and second toes, a half thumb-width in front of the base joint of the big toe. It continues in the groove between the metatarsal bones of the first and second toes to reach Liver 3, which can be found in a depression at a distance of one and half thumb-widths from the base joint of the big toe. The meridian traverses the back of the foot to Liver 4, situated in a depression next to the clearly palpable tendon of the tibialis anterior and a thumb-width anterior to the medial malleolus.

From Liver 4, the meridian continues by crossing the inner border of the tibia and ascending in the direction of Spleen 6 (three thumb-widths above the medial malleolus). It then follows the inner border of the tibia upwards to Liver 6, seven thumb-widths above the medial malleolus. There it curves around the inner portion of the two-headed calf muscle (gastrocnemius) to course to the inner aspect of the knee, where, with the knee bent, Liver 8 can be located at the end of the knee crease, anterior to two distinctly palpable tendons (semitendinosus, semimembranosus). On the thigh, the meridian initially continues alongside these tendons, and then follows the adductors. The strongest tract of this muscle group defines the pathway of the liver meridian.

Above Liver 12 (one thumb-width below the upper border of the pubic bone and two and a half thumb-widths lateral to the body's midline), the meridian veers laterally. Starting at Liver 12, it crosses the groin and curves gently across the abdomen towards the chest. The next landmark is Liver 13, located at the free end of the eleventh rib. Coming from Liver 13, the meridian crosses the lower border of the ribcage and courses to Liver 14 in the sixth intercostal space, directly below the nipple.

Key Areas of the Liver Meridian

Feet and Hips

Like the spleen meridian, the liver meridian begins at the big toe. These two meridians are often in opposition to each other. The spleen meridian embodies our centre. The liver meridian can help us to find our centre, but it can also lead us away from it. If we follow plans that aren't congruent with our dreams and longings, we get further and further away from who we truly are, from ourselves, until we no longer know where we actually stand in life. This can result in tension and discontent, in inner pressure. Since pressure condenses energy, sooner or later pressure always leads to heat. Heat rises, upwards to the head. A red face, red eyes. We lose the ground beneath our feet. This is clearly visible in tension in the feet, and especially in the toes. The tendons become shorter, especially around Liver 2, *xing jian* or 'Moving Between', and Liver 3, *tai chong* or 'Great Surge'. Liver 2 is assigned to the fire element, Liver 3 to the earth. Rising fire, lack of traction on the ground. The big toe easily lifts up and we lose both our inner and outer stability. The liver dominates the spleen.

Costal Arch

The liver organ is situated below the right costal arch, and this is where we find two key points on the liver meridian: Liver 13, *zhang men* or 'Chapter Gate' or 'Gate of the Ordering', and Liver 14, *qi men* or 'Gate of Hope'. This area, too, expresses the conflict between the liver and the spleen meridians. Liver 13 is the alarm point of the spleen. Liver 14 is the alarm point of the liver. For the spleen, the alarm bells start ringing when our inner centre is threatened by too much pressure or too much pent-up aggression. When too many chapters or sections of our lives have not been completed. All the loose ends lead to stagnation. They tie up energy. They disturb the free flow. Taking a deep breath requires effort. There's tension in the diaphragm and in the flanks. The entire area feels tight and is sensitive to pressure. And often there is also a feeling of pressure in the chest.

This is a condition that makes it difficult to open the Gate of Hope to start a new cycle. There will be a state of alarm for the liver, whose life principle is about growth and development. Liver 14 is the last point of the body's energy cycle. From Liver 14, the energy flows once again to the lungs, so that a new cycle can begin at Lung 1. If the energy reaches Lung 1, there is hope since the life principle of the lungs is the big 'yes' to life.

The Liver Meridian: Key Points

- Associated element: Metal element
- Quality: Yin
- Time on the organ clock: 1am–3am
- Animal quality: Ox
- Partner meridian: Gallbladder meridian
- Twinned meridian: Pericardium meridian
- Opposite meridian: Small intestine meridian

Chapter 17

The Third Meridian Family: Pericardium, Triple Heater, Gallbladder and Liver

Self-Actualisation

The third meridian family is the last one to develop. If we compare our life plan to a tree, the roots, by ensuring our nourishment, represent the first meridian family. The trunk represents the second meridian family, providing stability, strength and clarity in the core of our being. And the branches, twigs and leaves, flowers and fruits symbolise the third meridian family, expressing the potential that has developed out of the seed. What we bring to this world becomes visible and tangible in the third meridian family. It comprises the meridians of the pericardium, triple heater, gallbladder and liver. It begins to evolve around the age of six, reaches a high point during puberty and consolidates during adulthood.

As the child starts school, communities beyond the family become increasingly more important. Social interaction, building friendships, looking for new roles in new groups – all this falls under the remit of the pericardium meridian. It also includes an increase in discovering sexual identity, experiencing oneself as a girl or a boy, recognising and being interested in differences. All this involves highly complex situations of learning and experiencing in which it is easy to lose one's bearing – or oneself. It's therefore no surprise that it's precisely in this life phase that the triple heater emerges as the guardian of our balance. It protects and integrates. And it provides a further important function: it opens and closes our 'outer' gate. In this developmental phase, the gate has to be closed quite frequently for processing and digesting, but also for creating some distance from the parents. The triple heater is like the door to the child's room which suddenly doesn't stay open any more. The prepubescent child wants to determine its life to a greater extent; he or she is striving for more independence. This process goes hand in hand with the gallbladder meridian coming into its own.

The gallbladder makes autonomous decisions, and it has the courage necessary to do so. It develops an awareness of the consequences of our actions, and it plays around with that. It questions rules and creates its own guidelines. This can lead to friction and arguments, to tantrums and rage, all of which are associated with the gallbladder meridian, but also with the liver meridian. The relationship to the world is changing. During the phases of the first and second meridian families, we experience ourselves as beings that depend on the world. With the development of the third meridian family, there is an awakening of the claim for designing our world according to our ideas. At this point, the liver meridian comes increasingly into play. It develops and experiments with ideas and visions, approaching them with the caution they're due. It designs the draft for its masterplan of life. The core task of the third meridian family is to take our place in the world, independently and congruent with our nature and our ideas. The central questions are as follows: How do I actually want to live my life? What are my dreams? How can I blossom to the fullest? The third meridian family corresponds to the fifth level of Maslow's pyramid of needs – self-actualisation.

Just like the other two meridian families, the third family also requires good support so that all its pertaining meridians can evolve freely. That's not exactly easy, as there will be many very intense changes and upheavals, and the growing child has to resolve many conflicts by and within itself. On the one hand, freedom beckons. On the other hand, the child needs a feeling of safety. It may be great to play it cool during the day, but at bedtime it's nice to get a hug. While we may have acquired a taste for autonomy, we are conscious of the ongoing dependency. And then, of course, there's the whole thing about sex and hormones. Often, body and mind go their separate ways. The physical form is already grown up, but the mind and spirit are not. Or vice versa. The balance continues to be fragile for a long time to come, and it doesn't take much for it to topple. It requires space that is as loving as it is big, and it requires trust, understanding and open protective arms always. It's about a young person's self-actualisation, about the balancing act between boundaries providing orientation and limitation on the one hand, and boundlessness without friction on the other.

Many crucial abilities and skills important to our further life path are moulded in this phase. The gallbladder has to learn to live with its decisions and deal with their consequences. The liver requires strength for believing in its dreams and developing its creative component. The pericardium meridian takes care of all interpersonal aspects. And the triple heater endows us with the gift of self-regulation.

As was the case with the second meridian family, the third family, too, depends on the developmental stages of its preceding meridians. The third meridian family, with pericardium (7pm to 9pm), triple heater (9pm to 11pm), gallbladder (11pm to 1am) and liver (1am to 3am), takes the last place in the organ clock. Let's return to the image of a tree. Without strong roots and a sturdy trunk, it is hardly conceivable that this tree could bear big and delicious fruit. The connection between the second and third meridian families is obvious: When no stable identity was developed during the former, how could the latter express anything? How could the liver develop its dreams when there is no substrate? Based on what kind of desires could the gallbladder make its decisions? How mature are we for deep relationships if we are riddled with insecurity and feelings of lack of self-worth?

Puberty often mirrors the developmental state of the meridians. It will always be a turbulent time but it can turn into a serious and dramatic phase when the third meridian family lacks its foundation. Then puberty will be dominated by chaos, aggression, anger, rebellion and a lack of orientation. A young person may end up shunted aside without ever having gained momentum. They may be unstable and prone to succumbing to older role models who are stuck in their own developmental loop. They lack motivation for orienting themselves towards the future. They may seek refuge in excessive behaviours to avoid all the problems mounting up.

The development of the third meridian family never reaches completion, and pubertal behavioural patterns drag on, even into old age.

In our work with meridians and meridian families, we assume that it is never too late to integrate those life principles that haven't fully developed yet. However, this requires a clear and radical stock-take and the search for the right button to push. While problems around aggression can be associated with the third meridian family, their roots can often be found in the first. Conversely, a person may have sufficient, even deep-reaching trust, but was never sufficiently challenged to train their decision-making muscle. That could be enough to cause a small dent in the wheel of life so that it can't run smoothly; clearly a problem located in the third meridian family, most likely in the gallbladder. Sometimes it's only one meridian that needs our focus and attention. Sometimes it's several. But let's be clear: there's no point replacing a few slates on the roof when the basement is about to collapse. In such cases, the meridian system offers us excellent guidance.

Chapter 18

How to Get Started

Just Begin!

This book can't replace professional treatment for more serious problems of either a physical, mental or emotional nature. In case of physical complaints, you should always see a medical doctor. The strength of TCM lies in prevention. Dealing with a disease before it even arises is obviously the best medicine. But assuming we can avoid ever getting ill is an illusion. Problems, suffering and death are all part of our life cycle. To return yet again to the image of the wheel of life mentioned at the beginning of the book: if the wheel is running smoothly, if we have regularly maintained its spokes, if everything is in balance, then we are much better placed to cope with the challenges and calamities life throws at us. However, when we are in a rough and uneven state, it doesn't take much to throw us off course, and larger obstacles are even worse to deal with. Now is the best time to begin!

Many of the connections between body, mind and spirit described in this book may appear a bit simplistic and banal. Can suppressed frustration really conjure up a headache? Can difficulties with decision making really result in gallstones? Can excessive rumination really lead to weak connective tissue? You don't have to believe any of that. TCM is a system of medicine rooted in practice and experience. All I'm asking is for you to come with an open mind and a non-judgemental attitude. Open your eyes and ears, look around you, listen. After 30 years of clinical experience, I have found the meridians to be full of life. In many cases, it was possible to significantly improve or completely alleviate physical complaints, sometimes of a severe nature, by following the exercises described in this book in conjunction with treating the meridians. The improvement on a physical level was often accompanied by intense and exciting personal growth – an important step towards overall wellbeing.

Changing behavioural patterns and lifelong habits is certainly not an easy task. A radical change of course requires much energy and willpower – precisely what many people are lacking. Otherwise, people wouldn't just be flirting with the idea of changing direction; they would have already done it. For this reason, I'd like to emphasise the importance of force of habit. I'm sure you're familiar with this concept. You decide it is about time to exercise more, you come up with an excellent exercise routine, you become a member of a gym, you book courses, and so on and so forth. And what happens next? The first week you're still fully motivated; every second day, you do one hour of high-intensity training. And what happens next? The following week – damn, something cropped up on Thursday. And on Saturday something prevented you going again. After three weeks you are plagued by a bad conscience rather than well-deserved sore muscles. Your plan is burning out, just like the fireworks on New Year's Eve, along with all your resolutions.

It's much better to trust the force of habit and the power of small steps. There's no excuse for not exercising ten minutes a day. No day can be so busy, chaotic or rough that you can't manage ten minutes. It's much easier to turn this daily ten minutes into a routine than a programme that is more challenging simply because it takes more time. Each routine creates a new habit. Exercise will become an integral part of your everyday life. After all, it's all the little habits that make up our life.

It is said that it takes about two months to establish new routines. This has to do with the neural networks in our brain. As creatures of habit, we are accustomed to giving preference to existing neuronal connections. We have a tendency to always use the same routes, even if, in the long term, they end in a cul-de-sac. Beating out new paths takes time and continuity. But once a new path has been established, it's much easier to walk on it. It's exactly the same with the exercises in this book: dedicating ten minutes every day to your personal development, working on it every day, is probably the best investment you can make in your health, growth and wellbeing.

More pronounced imbalances in the meridian system need external support. Give it a go and try the treatment options of TCM – acupuncture, herbal therapy or manual methods such as Shiatsu. You will be surprised how much this could change your life. May it run more smoothly!